CARE MANAGEMENT

WITHDRAWN

HEALTH AND SOCIAL CARE MANAGEMENT

A Guide to Self-development

Sara Whiteley BSc, PhD, RGN, RMN,
runs her own research and consultancy service in health and social care

Richard Ellis BSc, MEd, Cert Ed, LGSM, RSA (Dip TEFL),
is a consultant and provides training in communication skills

Sinclair Broomfield MA, Cert Ed,
is a consultant and provides training in the management of health care

FOREWORD
Professor Frank Clark CBE
General Manager, Lanarkshire Health Board

A member of the Hodder Headline Group
LONDON • SYDNEY • AUCKLAND

First published in Great Britain 1996 by
Arnold, a member of the Hodder Headline Group,
338 Euston Road, London NW1 3BH

Whilst the advice and information in this book is believed to be true and
accurate at the date of going to press, neither the authors nor the publisher
can accept any legal responsibility or liability for any errors or omissions
that may be made.

British Library Cataloguing in Publication Data
A catalogue record for this book is available from the British Library

Library of Congress Cataloging-in-Publication Data
A catalog record for this book is available from the Library of Congress

ISBN 0 340 61411 0

Typeset in 10/12 Palatino by York House Typographic Ltd, London
Printed and bound in Great Britain by J W Arrowsmith Ltd, Bristol

Contents

Foreword

When I was asked by the authors to write the Foreword to this book the title caused me to reflect on the need for such a publication at the present time. There is no doubt that health and social care continue to face a significant change of agenda, both in terms of pace and scale. In rising to the many challenges brought about by change, health and social care managers need to look to developing their own personal knowledge, skills and abilities. This publication is therefore timely and is particularly attuned to today's agenda.

The text is extremely well researched and although its comprehensiveness causes it to be lengthy, this should not deter the intending reader since the content is relevant to the current scene. The focus of the publication on health and social care settings ensures its topicality in a climate of change, and the well constructed and easy to read text retains the reader's interest. Whilst the range of key current topics covered is extensive, the stand-alone nature of each chapter enables the reader to 'dip in' to topics of special interest. However, the strength of the publication lies in its cohesiveness when taken as an entity in terms of both personal and technical development. The book is essentially a walk through the portfolio of skills required by managers in today's public sector, enabling a good appreciation of the elements of that portfolio, in theory, practice and context. The inclusion of a wide range of references and further reading materials will be useful to the reader interested in pursuing specific elements.

Whilst the book, when taken in its entirety, is a comprehensive reference on management development for middle managers, I would highlight as particularly important the sections of the text dealing with the issues of communications, leadership and team building. The importance of good communications within and between the health and social care settings cannot be over emphasized. Inextricably linked to good communications are the issues of leadership and team building. Leadership skills are an essential prerequisite to the management of change and will increasingly become a vital tool in the middle and senior managers' armoury if they are successfully to address the challenges facing health and social care. Whilst I referred above to the importance of managers looking to their own self-development, this is not to over emphasize this aspect since, ultimately, it will be the manager who can successfully lead and build a strong cohesive team with a corporate sense of purpose who will achieve success in the current climate of change. I would therefore exhort readers to dwell for a moment on the important messages contained in these sections and to think carefully about their relevance for their own work setting.

In an environment where there is a dearth of topical and relevant reference material for managers, the authors have produced a valuable text which contains very real messages for health and social care managers in the mid-1990s and beyond, and readers cannot feel other than challenged about their own state of development as managers.

FC

Acknowledgements

WEB Associates would like to thank members of staff at Dumfries Health, both the Acute and Community Trusts, who provided the original audience for much of this material as it was delivered in various courses. The many excellent projects that were delivered as a follow-up by participants on these courses provided stimulus to the writing of this book. Particular thanks to Richard Swift, Alice Drife and Kathy O'Reilly who assisted us with the organization and development of these courses.

WEB Associates are indebted to Professor Frank Clark and his colleagues at Lanarkshire Health Board for agreeing to write the Foreword and their suggestions on various chapters of the text.

We are particularly indebted to Robert Shirley, Consultant in Health Economics and Finance, for his expert assistance with the writing of the chapters on costing and budgets, also to Jeremy F. Cook, Deputy Director of Finance, Edinburgh Royal Infirmary for specialist advice on these aspects.

Thanks also to our panel of readers: Marie Cerinus, Carol Gortmans, Elaine Yardley, Jane Howell, Lora Green who very kindly gave of their time to suggest additions and deletions to us.

Especial thanks to spouses, partners and members of families: Hazel, Sally, Carol, Grace, Charles and Victoria for their support and for their helpful advice during the period of composition.

1

Introduction

The origins of this book lie in the courses that WEB Associates have been running for various health boards, NHS Trusts and other public sector organizations in Scotland, particularly for Dumfries Health. The courses entitled 'Self Development for Managers' are aimed at those staff who have been appointed to management positions such as G grade nurses, clinical directors and first line managers in social care. In other words, managers who still work directly with those who provide care to patients and clients, and often find themselves 'caught in the sandwich' between more senior managers making demands at an organizational level and 'shopfloor' colleagues who, despite everything, are trying to deliver a high quality service.

Many managers promoted to this level have had a professional training without much in the way of formal management training, and this means that to a large extent, 'learning by experience' takes place, particularly at first. In answer to the question then 'Why another book on management?' we would claim that this one is specifically geared to the needs of this group of staff in social care and the health service and does not purport to be a general text on the subject. Most importantly, it is a text geared towards people management, which is one of the more sensitive areas of management and one which, if worked at, can make life easier for all those who work within a manager's domain.

The contents of this book are derived from our collective, first-hand experience of working with, and for, those in front-line management situations. By combining theoretical knowledge with the practical, everyday experiences of the work situation, a great deal of material can be made available for use by a wider audience. This includes information and examples from participants of the 'Self Development for Managers' courses; material collected whilst carrying out audits and management consultancy in the public sector; books and journals which represent much in the way of current thinking on management; and finally anecdotal material from those on wards, in community care settings and in other voluntary or statutory sector settings. All of these sources provide a rich and varied commentary on managing in the public sector today.

Where is management going and what contribution does this book make?

During the last few years in the UK and in many other countries, management has been devolved downwards from senior to middle and from middle to junior levels. In fact in some organizations the team leader and supervisor is a manager in the sense that he or she has some power to spend money, and has some responsibility for staff training, appraisal, induction or supervision. Hence, we see power moving down from senior nursing staff to ward and team levels; we see budget holding passing down from a few accounts staff to supervisors and junior managers.

In order to manage at all, we need to manage ourselves. This book seeks to help managers to do this. The book is subtitled, 'A Guide to Self-development' for a good reason. We believe that we need to manage ourselves effectively before we can manage others. This introduction summarizes what we feel are the key aspects to both of these skills.

You may well have entered the health or social services through a professional training of some kind, as physiotherapist, social worker, doctor, nurse, probation officer, etc. You have been given management responsibilities. Now you may increasingly face a tension between being a *player*, i.e. carrying out *professional* duties and hands-on care with patients and clients, and being the *manager*. This is the archetypal player/manager dilemma.

Role clarification

One important way through this tension is to clarify exactly what you are supposed to be doing in both roles. So many managers in this position suffer unnecessary stress and tension because they fail to clarify with their line managers what their remit is as far as their professional 'hands-on' work with patients/clients is concerned, versus their managerial responsibilities.

Role blur is what happens when we are not clear what we are supposed to be doing. This can lead to a loss of confidence and, as we have said, increased stress. Furthermore, if we are not clear as to our respective roles, then presumably nor is our boss, our staff or our colleagues. This can lead to all kinds of problems.

As changes continue to occur in health and social care (as they most certainly will), precise boundaries between player and manager will be hard to pin down. However it is in our own, our staff and clients'/patients' interests to work at this clarification. Increasingly the manager role will become more predominant for many of you. The more effectively you can perform this the more time and energy you will have for the player role.

There is another aspect of self development that is important for you to consider, namely the fact that not only do you have to think about improving your skills so that those whom you manage will benefit from your increased expertise, but you also need to invest in your own future in terms of career development and possible promotion. Opportunities for developing careers in the public sector have decreased over recent years, as the number of management posts has steadily decreased. Words like 'rationalization' and 'down-sizing' may make us all smile ruefully, but the result of this is that there is more and more competition for fewer promoted posts.

Some of you reading this text will not necessarily wish to move higher up the tree, but concomitant with the reduction in management posts is the need for those still in the organization to take on more managerial responsibility. For either reason working to improve your management skills is a worthwhile investment of time.

What does this book contain?

Charles Handy has written widely about the management revolution and points out the trend for large organizations to settle down into smaller and smaller teams and units. He remarks upon the fact that if you examine the structure of many organizations all those neat lines of the typical hierarchical chart are being replaced by 'blobs' and amoeba-like patterns, as teams replace departments, project groups take the place of divisions and even meeting rooms become network rooms!

All this has increased the need for managers who are good at working with teams and who are in fact team builders and enhancers. We devote some time to this area, looking at *team building* and *handling groups*, as well as *delegation* and *motivation* skills. The whole area of *leadership* is considered and, crucially, the skills involved in successful *negotiation* are examined.

Underpinning any successful manager, or indeed any successful organization, time and time again the issue of *communication* arises. We mainly hear about, or stop to consider communication only when things have gone wrong. Ever turned up for a meeting that has been cancelled? Tried to telephone someone only to get lost in, or held up by an internal switchboard? Sent out an important memo that no one bothers to read and then people moan because they are not kept informed? Communications are crucial to the smooth running of an organization and as a manager you must both be 'good' at communicating, as well as managing your communications. Further, there is a general recognition that if organizations are going to remain responsive to the needs of their 'customers' (another idea which has gained currency) then there has to be a short-circuiting of layers of command and lines of communication. The pace of development in electronic communications, such as fax, e-mail, laptop computers and mobile phones, has made it possible as never before for senior managers to keep in touch with staff and to monitor how devolved budget holding, decision making and evaluation is proceeding. Because of the importance of communications, we have devoted two chapters to this topic and suggest that they are crucial reading for everyone (*see* Chapters 4 and 8).

Still part of this same revolution, whole swathes have been cut through management personnel. The banks, building societies and BT, to name but a few, have reduced the number of those managing by over 50 per cent in some cases. Those who have survived are finding themselves even busier, less secure and under increased pressure. All this is causing increased *stress* for middle and junior managers. Managers' roles have been widened, their responsibilities have been enlarged yet at the same time their existing (i.e. professional) work may only have been cut back a little.

Public sector organizations are no exception to these pressures and one of the most useful skills to learn in this situation is good *time management*. If you can organize yourself well, then there will be more time to spend organizing, helping and managing others. Conversely, the opposite is true. If you cannot manage your own time, then how can others be expected to take you seriously – assuming that they can catch up with you! Chapter 3 looks at time management and provides practical examples of how to start making the best of your time – never feel you need to join the 'lunch is for wimps' gang!

Three other issues that we have considered over the years to be of vital importance to the middle manager are addressed in this book. The first has already been mentioned in passing and relates to the important issues of *budgeting and finance*. This is probably the skill most far removed from anything that professional staff have addressed in training and education to date and for that reason alone we have dedicated two chapters to the subject. One deals with the subject of costing (Chapter 10). It is important to understand this concept before moving on to the next chapter on budgeting (Chapter 11), which is the part of the finance process that will probably be most relevant to you.

Secondly, monitoring has gained credence as never before and through formal appraisal, pay is often related to performance and terms of employment are increasingly altered from permanent to three year contracts or less. As a manager you need to know how to handle your own appraisal process, but more importantly you will be responsible for appraising and evaluating the staff for whom you have managerial responsibility. Yet skills in *appraisal* and *evaluation* can also be applied across other areas at work and we also take a look at these in order to help you to be able critically to evaluate your department and the work carried out by your staff.

The third and final element of this book – *quality assurance* – comes from the motivation to assure quality of service and the care that is delivered. It comes from the outside through contracts, charters and occupational standards as well as from within through professional standards and the need as a manager to look towards value for money.

Taking all of these issues into account, it is no wonder that there are many staff who yearn for former times when they knew their place in the line, knew clearly what had to be done and by when, knew they could always pass up difficult decisions and that they would not be blamed if something went wrong. No wonder then that there are some who would cheerfully cry: 'bring back Matron'. It is very unlikely that those days will return; devolving management downwards is likely to be an accelerating trend. This book aims to help you to cope.

Can anyone really make me a manager?

It is fair to say that there has been a long debate as to whether managers can be trained to become more effective. Some would say that it is only by doing the job, actually managing, that one can gain the necessary insights that go to improve management skills. Others say that only some have the necessary qualities that can make an effective manager – qualities of leadership and drive, etc. We shall be entering into this debate in this book. However, one only has to glance through the pages of most quality newspapers to see the number of advertisements for Masters in Business Administration, Diplomas in Management etc., that are being offered. Does this mean that managers can in fact be trained, or is it just that universities and private providers have found a good market and are seeking to exploit it for all it is worth?

Our aim in this text is to raise the awareness of management issues with you, the reader, to outline specific management skills and approaches with those who are, in fact, managing at the moment. It is important here, because of this aim, to spend some time considering how it is possible for you to continue to learn whilst carrying out your regular duties, especially if you do not have the opportunity to attend a training course or you wish to use this text in conjunction with a period of study. After all, we are aiming to enhance substantially your knowledge and expertise. It would be helpful for you to have some insight into how and why people learn, and to this end, the next section addresses this important issue.

Being able to practise what you are reading and reflect on your actions is of great value in developmental terms. In some ways you are in a much better position to benefit from this text because you are in fact on the job and not sitting in a lecture hall. You will be in a position to 'test out' the ideas and gauge their impact.

Learning from experience and learning styles

Most people would claim that they learn from experience, but let us just examine this idea further for a moment. In terms of your position as manager of a unit, ward or department, you have responsibility not only for your own learning, but to an extent, also that of your team. You therefore need to be able to recognize some of the different aspects of how people learn so that you will take as much as possible from this book, but also so that in the future you can help your staff to learn effectively. It is likely for all of you that most learning will take place through the workplace and your experiences at work; hence we need to examine the idea further.

Individual learning

In work situations, when we encounter a problem, our primary concern is likely to be to solve it and then get on with the next thing in our busy lives. So how and when does the learning from this happen, if at all?

Sometimes the experience has been so traumatic and far-reaching that we spend time reviewing and developing new guidelines or protocols, for example, to try to ensure that similar situations do not happen again – so that we *do* learn from experience. Thankfully, however, such events are probably rare for you. What about more everyday situations such as handling a difficult client or planning your work?

Understanding how to learn from experience is a very useful skill for the manager. Honey and Mumford (1988) provide a valuable insight into how we learn, or could learn, from experience. They suggest that learning from experience involves four different stages:

1. *Having the experience.* For most of us this means that events occur to us, i.e. we *react* to things that happen. However, you can also seek out experiences quite deliberately in a *proactive* way. Much work-based student activity is undertaken in this way so that the learner has experienced a range of 'planned' events and can reflect on them. Once we are outside the student role, to what extent do we try to seek out experiences with the deliberate intention of learning from them? Job secondment and job rotation are examples of this process at one level – and at another is the experience of opportunities such as joining a project team, undertaking a new procedure, or making a presentation when this is not part of your current range of competencies.

2. *Reflecting upon and reviewing the experience.* This is a process of going back over the experience (perhaps with a colleague or mentor) and reviewing what has happened without seeking to place any blame, and determining what you have learned, and if relevant how you can prevent such a problem happening again. Busy managers find it difficult to spend time reviewing, but the argument is that time invested now in learning from an event will be more than repaid by the improvement in handling which will follow from the learning. Thus, you will move from being an expert 'fire-fighter' to becoming a more effective strategist and thus reduce the number of 'fires' that need to be tackled.

3. *Drawing conclusions from the experience.* From the reviewing process, you will be able to draw conclusions – rather than jumping to conclusions. Thus it will take some time, involve careful scanning of the elements of the situation picked up at the review stage and should lead to specific and grounded conclusions.

4.   *Planning the next step.* From the conclusions arrived at, planning involves converting these into some plan for future activity and ensuring that the 'lessons learned' pay for themselves.

The extent to which you are currently performing in these stages will probably be related to your personal learning style preferences. Honey and Mumford (1988) identified four different learning styles as follows:

- *The activist.* Activists often seek out new situations and throw themselves enthusiastically into them. They find these exciting and enjoy the 'here and now' of doing things. They are action-oriented people who act without necessarily considering the consequences until later. For them, learning occurs mainly through 'doing'.
- *The reflector.* Reflectors like to stand back and observe what is happening and tend not to get too involved. They are cautious by nature and analytical in approach. In group situations they maintain a low profile. For them, learning occurs after they have had an opportunity to reflect on the experiences.
- *The theorist.* Theorists like to integrate their observations into well-established theoretical perspectives. They tend to think in a logical and step-by-step fashion and search for order and system. In terms of their experiences, learning occurs through the linkage between current events and logical systems.
- *The pragmatist.* Pragmatists are primarily concerned with trying out new ideas, techniques and theories to see if they work in practice. They like to get things done and test them in what they would call the 'real world'. They will absorb lots of ideas initially, but reject those which do not seem to work for them. Learning for them, therefore, comes from the application of theory to practice.

Most people tend to have one or two dominant or preferred styles and are less keen on the others. We all know of group training situations when the trainer announces an exercise following some input and there are a range of responses:

'Oh great, an exercise – when can we start?' (activist)
'I think I'll just sit this one out. Do you need an observer?' (reflector)
'Before we start, can you just give us the theoretical basis for this?' (theorist)
'I hope I can pick up a technique or two from this!' (pragmatist)

Of course, on reflection, you will appreciate that *all the styles* are appropriate at different stages in any learning cycle and that if some of the styles are less favourable for you, it is worth while trying to become more willing to try them out and actively enhance the experience for you. People can and do strengthen all their learning styles once they have understood the differences and their particular preferences.

In terms of this text, we have attempted, within the limitation of the written word, to offer a variety of different learning experiences, providing some exercises, encouraging reflection through the use of case studies, outlining some theory or logic as a basis for an approach, and through giving summaries or checklists of tips and techniques for you to try out. As you work through the text, try to become aware of your own learning styles and strengthen those which are not so preferred.

Your team and their learning

The key question for all managers is how to get a positive or reasonably positive attitude towards learning across to your staff. Staff in health and social care services will need to keep up with what is happening in their professional area and in the wider organizational and political scene. Here are some thoughts for you as a *manager of learning:*

- Remember you are a *model*. If staff see you reading, taking notes from an article, going to talks, etc., then that should have a positive impact, particularly as you are a channel of information concerning learning opportunities.
- You should set the *expectation* that anyone coming from a course or having read an interesting text etc. should communicate the key ideas to the rest of the staff. This can be in the form of a very short and informal presentation, or summary report which can be circulated.
- You have a *responsibility* for putting up information (or seeing that someone else does) on staff noticeboards about courses, conferences, in-house seminars, new books in the library, etc. Do not forget that most people these days get their information from television. Keep an eye open for programmes that relate to your work. There is a constant stream of documentaries and 'specials' relating to reforms and 'challenges' within health and social care.
- Put training, learning and staff development on the *agenda* so that during meetings these aspects get discussed.
- Hold such things as soup lunches: free soup and bread in exchange for an exchange of ideas on a subject: How can we do it better? How can we learn from what Sheila has told us about her course? In any care setting it is usually very difficult to get hold of all staff at any one time, however it is important to make the best use of what time there is when staff can gather. The important thing is that *we can all learn from each other;* each member of staff can contribute to the staff development programme.
- Invite one of your staff to hold a *teaching session*. So often 'insiders' are ignored in terms of their abilities to train. Not only can it be very good for morale but it sends a powerful message to the others: we can and should learn off each other.

- Invite someone into the ward, the department, etc. to speak to staff at a coffee break, to *demonstrate* some new piece of technology, some new procedure, etc.
- Press for a training and staff development *policy* in your organization. Press for information from your own manager on the training budget – who gets what, how and when?
- Through your informal discussions with staff and through the more formal channels of appraisal you can make sure that questions of training and learning are seen to be *of importance and of high priority*. It is no good any organization having a declared policy that 'staff development is taken seriously here', when no manager ever asks his or her staff about the state of their development.

Conclusion

Whether you feel that you need to start at page one and continue through to the bitter end, or would prefer to dip in and out of the various sections, perhaps even leaving some out altogether, you should find something to help you and to set you thinking. We trust that this book helps you in your management role and in preparing others for that challenge.

References and further reading

Honey P and Mumford A (1988) *Developing Top Managers*. Gower, Aldershot.
Handy C (1993) *Understanding Organisations*. Penguin, Harmondsworth.
Schon D A (1983) *The Reflective Practitioner*. Basic Books Inc., New York.

2

Introduction to management

This chapter provides you with an overview of management. We define what management is, provide advice on clarification of your role as 'player/manager', and consider such aspects as management of change, delegation and motivation, and customer care. We survey the work of various key thinkers on management and how their ideas can contribute towards your needs in management, and finally consider two important themes which are central to your management role – change and business planning.

Introduction

So much has been written and lectured on in terms of management in the last few years that we can only briefly summarize a few of the points of the key thinkers who have influenced this process (see 'Further reading' for more sources of information). The overview that we have put together, however, illustrates the type of thinking that we believe lies behind 'good' approaches to people management skills. By considering some of the seminal thinkers in this field and looking at the issues which drive a sound approach to management, we believe that a more thorough understanding of management practice can be achieved.

There are two major aspects of management at the heart of what you are expected to do and that affect how you can effectively plan and run your service. We have therefore included them in this overview as they underpin much of the information that is provided in the rest of the book. The first of these is the *management of change*; this is key to running a good service. It cannot be overstated that the one constant thing in life is change, and poor management of this issue can reduce your chances of ever becoming an effective – and respected – manager. Good change management will help not only yourself and the organization, but also your staff, for whom clarity and consistency of approach can make all the difference to their commitment to and enjoyment of work.

Business planning on the other hand is something that is of importance to you and your position within the organization. Without a clear picture of what your service is to achieve over the coming year and how you propose to achieve this, then you cannot hope to manage your service effectively. Alternatively if you have a good guide to planned service provision, then you will make more time for effective management and the development of the skills that are described in this text.

Management: a piece of PIE

PIE stands for Planning, Implementing and Evaluation. According to the work of Druker (1979), these are the key functions of all management, whether it is to do with the ward, the department, the unit, hospital or day centre.

Druker divides the *planning function* into two: the operational and the strategic. The operational is the short to medium term – fixing one's eyes on events within one's reach. Strategic is that planning which is for events on the horizon. In Malaysia, strategic planning is given the name 2020. This refers to the target year and also, cleverly, the kind of vision required. Your organization may not be so far sighted; a three year target may be in your sights. It is important to separate out these two approaches: the near targets and the further ones. If we have no targets to aim for how can we plan? How can we enthuse our staff and determine the resources necessary if we are never looking at the horizon but always peering round the doorway? If we limit our vision we will never be able to recognize the possible threats and opportunities that may be approaching.

When thinking of planning it might be helpful to think SMART in terms of setting your objectives.

- *S for simple.* Goals should be expressed in simple, clear terms that you and your staff can understand. All too often in our experience managers are asked to pass on plans which they themselves are not clear about and find difficult to explain to their staff. Watch the management jargon here; get it translated before you pass it on. Communication from the manager to the staff should be a bridge towards common understanding; all too often it acts as a barrier to it.
- *M for measurable.* The crucial question is how will we know when we have achieved our goals? There is a need to think about how they will be measured. Broadly speaking we can do this in either qualitative and/or quantitative terms. For example, budgets are increasingly being devolved within public service organizations and many managers are now having to take responsibility for managing a budget. Keeping within 5 per cent, plus or minus, is an example of a quantifiable measure. However this may

not reflect the *qualitative* aspects of the goals of managing the department; these are concerned with the quality of the delivery of the service to patients, clients and service users. Increasingly there is a move within the public sector in the UK for organizations to publish league tables of performance: schools and the number of examinations that pupils have passed; hospitals and how many patients have recovered within what period of time; the police and how many criminals have been caught. There have been numerous criticisms that such tables only measure the quantifiable and do not take on board the qualitative aspects. There is a search now on to produce more value-added measures. You may well be part of this search for better measures and more realistic standards. You will find Chapters 12 and 13 on quality and evaluation helpful in this search.

- *A for achievable.* When we are setting goals it is important to be realistic and to seek to negotiate what is possible within given resources. We will be looking at the skills of negotiation in Chapter 7. The difficulty is that one person's realism is another's impossibility. This is where it is essential to negotiate in order to achieve a 'win–win' situation for both parties.
- *R for resourced.* There are a number of resources which may be important here, but the major one is likely to be the staff, as they comprise by far the largest single resource that we have in the public sector. In general terms we can estimate that 75–85 per cent of all our costs will be staff salaries and wages and attendant costs to do with their calculation and payment.
- *T for trackable.* Goals are often set for a 12 month period. It is important for managers to be able to monitor and thus take action if necessary to reassess the goals or change the order of priorities so that these have a chance of being realized. It is of little value to a manager to know that two years ago, for example, the unit was 18 per cent over budget. To be able to manage effectively, the manager needs information on a relatively *regular* basis so that actual performance can be tracked against planned perform- ance toward achievement of the goal. It is not good enough to be battening down the organization's hatches for the approaching financial hurricane; a warning of its approach should have been given earlier so that all the staff could get themselves prepared.

Next in PIE comes the *implementation* stage: the action. We show various approaches to this in Chapter 6. Essentially, after careful planning (and after consulting fully with colleagues and staff) the time comes for implementa- tion. However, the crucial point here is that good managers do not forget the E of PIE, that is the evaluation or review stage. It is not enough for the manager to act; he or she must be prepared to evaluate as they go along so that errors can be eliminated and, very importantly, lessons learned from success and from failure. Far too often we find that it is only when a failure occurs that managers try to learn from what happened. This can easily create a blame culture which can inhibit staff from ever taking risks. We need to be able to study our successes so that we can repeat and even better them, and we need to be able to reflect positively on failure so that really useful lessons can be learned.

We mentioned in our introduction the importance of managers being able to reflect on their experience. Evaluation is part and parcel of this process of thinking back to performance, establishing where changes will need to be made and so on. As the public sector increasingly comes under pressure for standards to be set for customer care and delivery of services, so it is increasingly important that managers are able to undertake thorough and illuminating evaluations of present practice. It is also important that lessons learned are disseminated to staff and colleagues and not left to gather dust in files.

Different roles

We have already seen just how important it is to clarify your role with respect to the player/manager dilemma. Minzberg (1973), another influential writer on management, suggests that managers should consider it essential to be prepared to play a number of roles in their work. The roles he lists include:

- leader of the team;
- administrator;
- conflict-handler and innovator.

The important thing here is that managers increasingly have to be versatile in their approach and be prepared to adopt more than one role. The British Institute of Management suggest that many modern managers are still riding their 'three speed bicycles', unaware that modern bikes have twenty and more speeds to offer. Thus managers need to be increasingly more flexible in their approach to situations.

Styles of management

We will be examining various aspects of this need for versatility in our chapters on communication and leadership and team building. We suggest that effective management relies on awareness that different situations require different styles. If you see a fire then you do not sit around organizing discussion groups and asking staff to carry out detailed reviews of fire risk management, you put the fire out, ask a member of staff to help, and see that it is properly extinguished. That is the *direct style*. However, after the fire has been put out and everyone is safe, then comes the time for discussion and analysis, for the revision of fire procedures and so on. In other words the manager is now using a more *collaborative style*.

Gods of management

Charles Handy (1991), has written that we can see organizational typology, that is the way that organizations group themselves together, as, amongst others, Zeus and Athena types. Those of you with longer memories of the health or social care services may well think that you used to work in a clearly Zeus structure, in which managers spent their time above the mere 'mortals' watching them from a distance and sending the odd lightning flash or thunderbolt to remind them of their all-seeing, all-knowing presence. Now with directorates and devolved management in health and social services there is more of the Athena (a goddess who listens and actually comes down from the heights), more of a collaborative approach, less of a rigid hierarchy. This has clear implications for management and its relationship with staff.

Delegation and motivation

These are two very important aspects of modern management, very much brought to the forefront by the move to devolved management in the public sector. We examine this aspect in Chapter 14 and in our discussion of time management. Delegation is about *letting go*. Managers increasingly have to recognize that they cannot do everything and one of the key management skills is the ability to delegate work to others, but in such a way that it is not seen as 'dumping'. Delegation is also about providing job enrichment and challenge to colleagues and subordinates. It is perhaps one of the most rewarding aspects of being a manager that you can act as a staff developer, delegating the appropriate and challenging job to someone else, guiding and coaching that member of staff through into a successful completion of the task. This aspect of the job also helps in the motivation of staff – another key aspect of management.

Managers have to plan for delegation; it cannot just happen or be left to whim. A time scale has to be agreed between the manager and the person to whom the work is to be delegated. Above all it has to be real delegation not the kind where the manager perches on the shoulder of a staff member and constantly watches what is being done; that is akin to smothering. Real delegation is 'hands off but both eyes wide open' It means keeping in touch with the person one has delegated work to and not just letting them get on with the job. The problem with this approach is that if there is a failure then the person who has had work delegated to is most likely get the blame and then the manager says 'Well I told you so. I knew I'd be better doing it myself – at least I'd then know it would get done.'

We have said that *motivating staff* is a key function of management. Managers need to care for their staff and one form of that care is the time they give to motivate them. By this we do not mean pushing them and demanding they work harder. Nor do we mean restrictive and coercive motivation, based on failure, fear of punishment and fear of loss of face. Motivation is about listening to staff, their needs, their hopes, providing them with encouragement and support, providing a gentle push where necessary and negotiating with them plans for job enrichment, staff development and training, secondment, job sharing. Managers increasingly have to create a climate and conditions in which staff are motivated constructively; replacing the 'I have to', with 'I want to and choose to'.

Customer care

This is an aspect of management that has come very much to the fore in recent years. Tom Peters (1988) and other writers have constantly preached the need for managers to know their customers. Although in the health and social services the word 'customer' may not be one that springs to our lips, the concept behind it is important. Our health and social care institutions are there for the customer. Increasingly in the UK with the development of the purchaser/provider split – that is where a health board/social work department is purchasing from a number of local and possibly not so local provider hospitals/social work centres – customer satisfaction measures will be taken into account when it comes to the settlement of contracts between the two. Peters also emphasizes the need for the manager to *care* for staff. We will see when we examine aspects of leadership and team building that this ingredient is crucial, especially during periods of very rapid and far reaching change.

The manager of change

There will be many references in this book to the problems and challenges of change. Increasingly in public service where change has come rather unexpectedly for many staff (after all, change is what has traditionally happened in the private sector, to coal fields, shipyards and motor car manufacturers, but not to us in the public sector), this lack of readiness for change and in many cases an unwillingness to change has made the role of management very difficult. The crucial management challenge is to take the staff with us through the change, rather than achieving change but with numerous casualties amongst the staff in terms of bitterness and loss of confidence. Most of you reading this book will only be able to influence change within your place of work; others will be in a position to fully manage the process.

Change is often experienced as a negative; for example you may hear the complaint 'Not another change – but we've only just got used to the last one!' Peters (1988) argues that innovation and change is at the heart of successful organizations and effective management, and far from being a negative force it is actually what drives the organization forward to bigger and better things. If you want to provide the best service you can then, you have to be constantly looking for different ways of doing it – *thus change becomes a constant.*

Management of change

We advocate a 'planned change' approach, which involves a series of stages all of which have implications for your broader management style, for example your approach to leadership and communication. The stages are presented and discussed below.

Stage one – creating the climate for change

Change starts with a recognition by you, or by the circumstances in which you work that a change is desirable or necessary. At the beginning of the change process, you will often find that your job as manager is to create a 'concern' as an indication or signal that change is necessary. The basis of this stage is your ability to create a degree of dissatisfaction within the status quo, in a nutshell, why should we change? Reasons for change within health and social services can be because *it can be done better* (quality), *quicker* (time saving), *more easily* (systems change, e.g. technology), *cheaper* (reduce costs) or *more accurately* (efficiency).

   Whatever the reasons at this stage, the manager is often trying to 'de-stabilize' the current position and thus lay the groundwork for change to begin.

   The manager should spend time talking to people and creating a ground-swell of shared concern about the need to change. This can also be thought of as a process of setting the agenda, thus avoiding the introduction of sudden change which can prove very difficult for certain individuals involved.

Stage two – getting people involved

Once the need for change has been established, it is important for the manager to identify the individuals who are most involved in and affected by the change. These are the *key players*, who are likely to be those who can ensure that the change takes place effectively. Communication with the key players and identifying the likely problems that the changes will bring, are the key issues at this stage. By identifying and seeking to solve problems before implementation of the changes themselves, the wise manager tries to avoid the pitfalls of introducing change quickly and spending a long time sorting out the problems that the speed of change has created. The other main advantage of this approach is that it involves the key players in the planning approach itself, so that they feel they have some commitment to the changes involved. For example, if we are asked to undertake a 3 per cent 'efficiency saving', then it is often more effective to involve those who will be affected by this in the planning and decision making about how it will be achieved. Imposed change of this kind can thus become at least managed by those whom it affects, avoiding feelings of helplessness.

Stage three – individual responses to change

As the change is beginning to be recognized more clearly, it is important for the manager to have an understanding of individual reactions to change that are likely to be encountered.

Comfort zones

We all tend to have a clear picture of ourselves in terms of what we are able to achieve – a self image which confirms our talents, skills and competencies. As long as what we are undertaking fits with this mind's eye picture of ourselves then we can generally cope. This is called our 'comfort zone', the perception of what we are capable of doing; we have become familiar and comfortable with ourselves and the activities in which we are involved.

As soon as we are encouraged to work outside our comfort zone, however, we feel 'out of place' and may experience anxiety and even stress and will need support and development to build a revised 'comfort zone' which will eventually incorporate a perception of the new competencies. However, the transition stage has to be managed and is likely to prove the main source of resistance to change – we like our comfort zone and want to stay there.

With the increase in devolved management, many first-line managers are being asked to take on new responsibilities for a range of areas previously undertaken by more senior managers. These new responsibilities may include attending meetings, presenting cases or preparing reports – areas outside the former experience and training of, say, many clinical staff and therefore outside their comfort zone. Comments such as 'I'm no good at these things' are commonly expressed.

Clearly what is needed is help and support through training and experience, but this is only possible when a person sees the importance of becoming competent in the area involved and is willing to move out of their original comfort zone.

To throw some light on this area, it is useful to think of change as involving an experience of loss – at least in the first instance. If we think of the reactions people have to more extreme examples of loss, such as bereavement, unemployment, loss of mobility and so on, we can identify a series of steps that people typically go through:

- *Denial.* This is an effective way of dealing with loss in the short term. Basically the person pretends/believes that the change is not going to happen. This 'head in the sand' strategy is very effective in protecting the individual from what may be experienced as a threatening change. For example, the introduction of new technology and the need for staff to learn new skills in handling computers can effectively be dealt with from an individual's point of view by a process of denial: 'I don't have to change, it is only happening in other parts of the organization'. The manager faced with denial in a member of staff may have to spend time preparing the individual for change, explaining and training so that denial becomes an inappropriate strategy.

- *Resistance.* Managers often report that resistance to change is quite strong amongst a relatively small number of individuals affected by the change. Nevertheless this small group can take up a disproportionate amount of the manager's time. One note of optimism about this is that if a member of staff is resisting change at least you know that the change has been recognized by this individual and that he or she is seeking to deal with it. Thus if a person is resisting the change and offering all sorts of reasons why it is not possible, then the manager has something to work with. Involving individuals as early as possible in the change process is probably the major way of helping to identify and overcome resistance before it becomes a major stumbling block. Providing explanations *and* helping people to see the benefits of change for them and the service are also strong ways of helping to overcome resistance. The key management style is to encourage expressions of resistance and acceptance of people's perceptions, fears and concerns and then to address these in a systematic way. No matter how enthusiastic you are about the change personally, always accept and listen to any individual's expression of concern.

  There is also the issue of a 'critical mass'. Once a significant number of people involved in the change in an organization have begun to work with it, this will support and encourage those who are more resistant to 'come on board' to follow suit. 'If it's alright for them, it must be alright for us.' One way to achieve this critical mass effect is to ensure that training is carried out for all those affected, thus creating a change climate which will move the group along.

- *Exploration.* At this stage, individuals are beginning to explore the implications of the impending change for themselves and the service. It is the beginning of a more optimistic phase and people need good leadership to help them make such an exploration and contribute to the way in which the change will ultimately be implemented. This is discussed more fully in Chapter 2. Use of techniques such as SWOT analysis in group discussions becomes a useful device to help individuals through this stage. As before, explanations and communication are vital to keep people informed of what is happening and thus reduce uncertainty. The team can be an extremely valuable source of both problem identification and ideas for solutions, and this team involvement further commits individuals to the achievement of successful change.

- *Commitment.* This final stage occurs when people are seen to be working closely together, where there is co-operation and better co-ordination in dealing with work matters. During the commitment stage it is possible to begin to set longer term goals, to build the team more fully and to start acknowledging and rewarding those individuals who are responding to change.

Stage Four – training, development and further communication

At this stage the manager is concerned with identifying specific training needs, areas of organizational development and above all the means and methods of communication to be used to keep people fully informed. In the light of the reactions to change, offering systematic support through coaching and training will help to alleviate much of the concern which may be expressed by those who have to learn new skills, adopt new systems or develop different strategies for dealing with the new agenda.

Some recent examples of change agenda requiring such development in the public sector include purchaser/provider relationship, negotiating skills, marketing and customer care, business planning and new technology. All of these are likely to involve learning new skills and developing new ways of doing things. The investment in such training and development is vital if major change is to be implemented effectively.

Stage five – getting it done, but building in a review

This is the final stage and involves the implementation and review of the changes themselves. During the implementation stage it is important to build in a series of reviews that allow you as manager and others who are affected by the change to take stock and evaluate the impact of the change. It is often difficult to predict all of the implications of change before it has been tried out. Thus a built-in review provides a safety net for further modification in the light of actual experience. Failure to build in review can, at an individual level, lead to a sense of helplessness; this is avoided if individuals know that at some point the whole process will be reflected upon and a refining can take place.

This short introduction to managing change should also take into account other aspects of the manager's role which are discussed elsewhere in the book: leadership and team building (Chapter 6); coaching and supporting (Chapter 14); and communication (Chapter 8).

Business planning

Increasingly, managers working in the public sector are being asked to contribute to a business planning process or in some cases actually writing business plans for their particular part of the service. A business plan is essentially a systematic statement about your aims and objectives and activities for – usually – the next 12 months. It needs to include details about what you intend to undertake and how you are going to do it, i.e. what staffing, premises, equipment and funding you need, plus reference to the marketing and monitoring of your proposed activity, including quality assurance.

The purpose of the business plan is to provide a major planning framework for your service over a given period of time. It ensures that you have thought through what resources you require and mechanisms for monitoring how well you are on target. It also indicates how your plan 'fits in' to the overall plan for the organization and provides a useful basis for discussing objectives with your staff.

What it involves

The business planning cycle consists of determining:

- where you are now with your service provision;
- where you want to be with this provision in the next 12 months;
- how you are going to get there; and
- how you will know that you have achieved what you said you would achieve.

Where you are now

To begin the process you need to review where you are at present and what organizational, legal and demographic factors you need to take into account in planning your service provision. Consider the following questions in relation to your current services.

- What do you currently provide?
- To whom do you provide them?
- What people, premises, equipment, support services and management arrangements do you have?
- What interdependencies do you have, e.g. with other agencies, on whom your provision relies?
- Who are the main interested parties, do they need to be consulted about the nature of the service you provide?

Where you want to be

To begin to determine where you want to be, you have to look at a number of organizational and generic factors which may influence the way in which your service will develop. The following checklist provides a summary of some of these factors.

- Demographic and epidemiological trends. What are the likely patterns you can discern over the next 12 months which will affect your provision of service?

- Changes in technology, e.g. information systems, new procedures
- Legal changes, e.g. Community Care Act
- National trends
- Organizational aims and objectives.

How you are going to get there

To consider how to get there, you need to include:

- Service objectives – maintenance and developmental
- Activities – possibly on a month-by-month basis
- Resources
- Marketing
- Management and staffing including staff development
- Development plans
- Financial implications
- Quality assurance – standards and mechanisms for monitoring.

How you will know what you have achieved

To determine whether or not you are achieving your planned targets you will need:

- regular management information on activity levels and actual financial positions, preferably on a monthly basis;
- regular quality feedback, e.g. through audit mechanisms, from customers;
- review of actual performance against the business plan, say on a quarterly basis.

The purpose of this monitoring activity is to enhance your ability as a manager to keep track of your service activity so that you can recognize, for example, when activity is not meeting the planned level, or resources are out of step with demands. You can then seek to take action earlier rather than later to correct the situation. Thus the plan becomes a proactive management aid.

Once you have undertaken the business planning process and followed the plan for a year, it is obviously going to be easier to do next time around, although you should avoid the trap of simply reproducing the same plan whilst allowing for inflation for the next year. You will need to use the checklists again to make sure that you take account of what are, inevitably, rapidly changing circumstances.

We hope this brief introduction has reassured you that business planning, far from being a theoretical exercise, can actually be an extremely valuable way of identifying your service provision plans and also the basis for negotiating developments in a planned and systematic way within your organization as well as helping you to manage the service more effectively.

Conclusion

We have presented here some of the key aspects to management. You could say that it has been a brief helicopter ride. In the following chapters, however, we will go into more detail on all the issues that have been raised. Remember to bear in mind the application of the skills that we are about to describe when you think of the two key processes of good management – change and business planning. How you deal with these two issues will depend on how you see yourself as a team builder, communicator, leader, etc.

We trust that the ensuing helicopter ride is not too bumpy or alarming – and that you land safely on the other side, or get back to where you started unscathed!

Further reading

Druker P (1979) *Management*. Pan Books, London.
Handy C (1991) *Gods of Management*. Century Business, London.
Minzberg H (1973) *The Nature of Managerial Work*. Harper & Row, New York.
Oldcorn R (1989) *Management*. Macmillan Education, London.
Peters T (1988) *Thriving on Chaos*. Pan Books, London.
Peters T and Austin T (1985) *A Passion for Excellence*. HarperCollins, London.
Scott C D and Jaffe D T (1990) *Managing Organizational Change*. Kogan Page, London.

3

Time management

In this chapter, we deal with the important area of time management. Increasingly, middle managers are required to take on more responsibility – through devolved management – and can perhaps no longer rely on existing practices to get them through a typical working week. By examining time management we offer a range of principles and practices which are intended to help improve your use of your most precious resource – time.

Introduction

Managing your time at work is about making the most effective and efficient use of your most precious resource in order to achieve your key goals. Within health care and social work as we have seen, anything from 70 per cent to 80 per cent of total spending is on staff. It follows that the way we use this resource is crucial.

Efficient use of time means undertaking an activity in the simplest, easiest and/or quickest way in order to reach the standards you want whilst achieving your aims.

But really before we decide the most *efficient* way to do something, we ought to decide if it is *effective*. Effective use of time means undertaking the activities that you *should* be doing. It follows therefore that you have to start by saying: 'Is this an effective use of my time?' and, if it is then use the time as efficiently as you can.

Having a clear picture of your job purpose generally provides the basis for determining those areas of your work on which you need to spend most time (see Case study 3.1).

Case study 3.1

> The manager of a social work department finds the secretarial support too overloaded to deal quickly with her letters to external agencies. To compensate for this she prepares her correspondence on her personal computer. Whilst her skills are quite good (and she enjoys doing it!) she realizes that a more effective use of her time would be to tackle the problem of the overstretched secretaries and thus solve the underlying issue. This is a much more *effective* use of her time.

In this chapter principles of time management are explored and practical ways to improve your use of time are offered.

What do you need to manage your time more effectively?

In order to manage your time more effectively, you need to:

- raise awareness of how you currently use your time;
- establish your goals, ask the question 'What am I employed to achieve?';
- determine your priorities – how important is the activity in relation to meeting your goals;
- plan your use of time;
- get organized, examine your habits and decide what you want to change;
- look at how you help (or hinder) your staff in their use of time; and
- be prepared to *negotiate* with your boss and your colleagues in order to achieve a better use of your time.

Why should I spend time trying to manage my time?

A number of benefits can be achieved through actively trying to manage your time:

- You can be more in control of how you use your time rather than everyone else determining how your time will be spent.
- You can reduce pressure, particularly when faced with deadlines or a heavy schedule.
- You can focus your work on the important things and thus achieve more in relation to the main reason for your employment.

- You can feel better about yourself because you are using your potential to the full.
- You should be able to achieve a better balance between time spent working and time spent at home, in leisure, etc.

Find out how you currently spend your time

Keep a time log

The first and most important step in taking more control of how you spend your time is to develop a picture of how you currently use your time. Many managers will argue that of course they know how they spend their time, but experience suggests that a real understanding and insight only comes about after a time log has been kept covering say two or three days and the manager really begins to see how the time is spent at present.

Keeping a time log is simple. Every fifteen minutes jot down what you are doing. Keep it simple, for example, travel to work, dealing with mail, phone call to John, meeting with boss, visiting a patient, and so on.

Keep the time log for at least two or three days, because we all know there is no such thing as a 'typical' day. Use a dictating machine if this is possible. Keep the log to cover your working day from the point where you leave home to the point when you return home, and if you take work home, remember to include that as well.

The purpose of this log is to give you a database so that you know how you currently spend your time.

Evaluate the results

The next step is to analyse this information. The following checklist provides some key questions to help you in this analysis:

- Did I do everything that I needed to do each day?
- Did I have enough time to do what I wanted to do?
- How did I actually spend my time? Develop some categories such as attending meetings, travel time, individual work, answering the telephone, visitors, personal breaks (e.g. coffee, lunch) – and become aware of what balance of your working day tends to be spent in each category.
- How much of my day did I have control of, and how much was determined by other people's demands?
- When was I most productive and when was I least productive?

Identify the changes you need to make

The final step is to identify changes that you need to make. If you are not satisfied with any aspects of the way you now know you used your time, then identify:

- activities you undertook that were of little benefit or value – not achieving your job purpose;
- specific problems that kept you from using your time well, e.g. interruptions, phone calls, unexpected problems occurring and so on;
- personal behaviour on your part that made it difficult to use your time wisely, such as procrastination, too much socializing and not being clear about your priorities.

Take a look at Case study 3.2.

Case study 3.2

Jean is a team leader in a community nursing setting and has seven staff of various grades reporting to her. She decides to undertake a time log over a three day period and, as she is both a manager and a player, i.e. she undertakes a case load which involves car travel in a rural area, she decided to use a portable dictating machine (but not when she was driving) and spoke into this about every fifteen minutes to capture what she was actually doing.

A number of very significant findings struck her when she reflected on the results of her time log:

- She became acutely aware that for two of the three days she failed to complete management tasks in her working day and spent a total of four hours working in the evening to catch up with these!
- She believes in a management style of 'open door' and found in her time log that staff were indeed very willing to come to her door and seek her advice and guidance on aspects of their work. She realized that a number of her staff were not clear as to the detail of their roles and were seeking to clarify these in these very short interruptions (including one in the car park as she was rushing off to see a patient!)
- As the team leader, she held a number of meetings with her staff, but they tended to ramble on, were not very structured (no agendas) and, while very sociable, seldom produced tangible outcomes and appeared to be a questionable use of her own and her staff's time.

As a result of this, she made a number of changes to the way in which she used her time:

- Over a three week period, she met with each of her staff on a one-to-one basis for an hour and clarified the roles she expected staff to undertake. She was surprised to find how much role-blur existed and both she and her staff benefited greatly from this clarification. It also meant that they had to consult her less than before, although they still checked out with her on issues which were particularly important.

- She decided to allocate a half day a week in her diary specifically for the purpose of undertaking important managerial work. When appointed as a team leader, she thought she could cope by just 'fitting things in', but her time log showed the inefficiency of this approach and by allocating space in her working week, she could focus her mind specifically on management activities.
- She undertook to improve meetings by doing a number of things. First, she indicated both a start *and* a finish time for the meeting and stuck to it (generally her weekly meetings were half an hour but they often over-ran).

  Secondly, she began to identify an agenda for each meeting and circulated it in advance of the meeting to ensure that everyone knew why they were meeting and what would be discussed that day.

  Lastly, she arranged for telephones to be redirected during the meeting time and for a notice to be put on the door saying 'Meeting in progress' as she discovered that in a busy practice, meetings were typically interrupted by staff who knew that all the nurses were in one room.

  Jean also decided to ask all her staff to undertake a similar time log and discuss the results as part of her weekly meeting.

Establishing your goals

Do you know what you are here to achieve – your purpose?

Managing your time is a lot easier once you decide what you want to achieve. This can be developed at a number of levels. Within organizations, we would start with the purpose of the organization so that ultimately we can see how our job fits in. The organization's goals become reflected in department or section goals – increasingly in the form of 'business plans' (as we saw in Chapter 2) in the public sector. These set out what the department or section intends to undertake in the work activity for the next 12 month period.

If both these organization-wide and departmental goals are fairly clear to you, then it becomes easier to identify your own job goals.

If, on the other hand, you are not too clear about these, then *a discussion with your line manager* and a reference to any planning documents in your organization will help to paint the 'big picture' within which you are going to undertake your own goal setting.

Another potential and major source of goals is some form of career review, appraisal or performance management scheme, increasingly used within organizations, and if such a scheme is in operation at present, then you may well already have a set of goals for, say, the next 6–12 months within which you can then determine your own use of time.

Whatever the schemes and information that you have available, some practical tips in effective goals setting that you might find useful are given in the SMART approach discussed earlier (page 11).

Thinking about goal setting can be applied to planning at all levels, e.g. the work of a single day, a week, a month or a year. Thinking back to the time log, it is a good discipline to apply SMART approaches to what you tried to achieve, i.e. your *goals* for that day.

Activity

If do not already have a set of goals for your job, consider having a discussion with your line manager to clarify your goals for the next 3–6 months. Think in terms of your key areas of activity within which you want to achieve a number of things and use this as the basis of your discussion.

Determining your priorities

'If you don't determine priorities for yourself, there are plenty of people at work who will do it for you!' Once you know what your goals are, then you can decide your priorities. Most managers would identify that in a busy working day they will undertake a range of activities, some of which are very important to their purpose, for example writing a report, presenting a case for improvement of some aspects of their service, but quite a bit of time can also be spent dealing with what might be called relatively trivial work.

One useful way to help identify priorities is to distinguish between *important* work and *urgent* work. According to the Pareto Principle we tend to spend 80 per cent of our time on 20 per cent of our work.

Important work is work that is going to contribute considerably to the achievement of your goals and therefore should get a higher proportion of your working time. Urgent work is work that is required to be done now but that, quite often, someone else has asked for and is not so important to you. Nevertheless, you are subjected to the urgency of this work by the insistence with which it is presented to you.

Urgent work, particularly of the trivial kind, is best dealt with first and quickly. This is why time management techniques often stress the importance of developing routines which allow you to handle this type of work quickly and efficiently, thus leaving you time to get on with the important work.

For example, allocate 20 minutes every day to opening and reacting to the mail that has come in. Much of this will involve quick answers, delegation and re-direction and can be dealt with straight away. However, if you leave it unresolved, incoming mail has a tendency to become a source of time wasting, as people start to telephone or stop you in the corridor to get the answers they are looking for.

Sometimes, work is both urgent and important and if this is so, clearly this must be given the highest priority, i.e. it must be completed first and you must spent a long time on it.

The important point is to have some system by which you can determine your priorities in an appropriate way; and while responding to the demands and needs of others in the organization, you need to protect time in your working day to focus your attention on those activities which will enable you to achieve your own goals (*see* Case study 3.3).

Case study 3.3

> A nurse manager recognized that because he worked in an open plan setting, people would drop in to see him or colleagues sitting a few desks away would see that he was free and 'pop over to have a word'. To protect some time in his working day to carry out important work, e.g. to prepare a paper on budget allocations, he had to develop some system of signalling that he did not wish to be disturbed. As he had recently been on holiday in Moscow where he had bought himself a distinctive Cossack hat, he decided to put this hat on as a signal that he did not wish to be disturbed and take it off when he was quite willing to be interrupted! After a few weeks of this, he realized how successful he had been when he heard his boss saying, 'Oh, sorry Bryan I didn't know you were busy, I will come back later'!

Planning ahead

Time spent planning is very wisely spent – it will save you lots of time later. Busy managers often find it very difficult to find time to plan what they are going to do. The picture of the manager who spends a lot of time reacting to demands and rushing around 'putting out fires' is unfortunately all too familiar. Taking some time to plan is the key to trying to deal with a short term crisis by tackling the underlying causes and effecting changes so that the amount of 'fire-fighting' actually reduces. Handling crises and working at fever pitch can be exciting to some people but to others can be stressful. With good planning, you should be better able to handle problems quickly, make decisions more effectively and avoid getting bogged down in day-to-day routine tasks.

Some tips on good planning

- Get into the habit of making a daily and weekly list of tasks that need to be done and put it in your diary. This can be done at the end of the working day – thus avoiding anxiety about what you have to try to achieve the next day – or first thing in the morning before you get directly involved in the day's activities.

- Prioritize your task using a system like the important/urgent split.
- Assess how long you intend to spend on each of the activities, remembering to spend more time on the important tasks and less time on the urgent ones, but perhaps sequencing them so that urgent ones are dealt with early.
- Allow for interruptions. No working day is free from unplanned events. If you review a number of days using the time log approach you can often identify patterns of interruptions and turn them into planned time.
- Schedule your work tasks in your diary. Be realistic and only schedule work for that day which you believe to be SMART, i.e. which is reasonable and for which you have sufficient time and effort.
- Keep your eye on the 'big' picture, i.e. your longer term goals. Use year planners on the wall to identify deadlines and other regular activities, e.g. monthly staff meetings, which may require some input from you in terms of preparation.
- In a typical working day, there will be times when you will feel that the work you are undertaking is highly productive but there will also be times when you feel it is a struggle to actually get started. Recognize that we all have different times of the day when we are more productive and less productive. Try to plan your more important work during the time when you are more likely to be productive and keep your more routine tasks for your less productive times.
- When faced with major projects and relatively long periods of time in which to complete them it is tempting to put off starting or simply to say to oneself 'well, I've got plenty of time for that.' Good planning of substantial projects involves breaking them down into a series of short term activities with a series of deadlines. Thus as each smaller part is completed, each builds towards the completion of the whole project.

Question 'How do you eat an elephant?'; answer 'A little bit at a time!'

- Remain flexible. Inevitably, things crop up which are entirely unpredictable and it is important to be willing to re-prioritize and change your schedule to meet the new demands. In such situations, taking a few minutes to think through your plan is well worth doing.
- Lastly, many managers undertake both a player and manager role as referred to in Chapter 1. For example, you may have management responsibility for a section, but part of your time is spent undertaking a professional responsibility as part of that team. The dilemma for such managers is deciding on the balance of time spent 'as manager' compared with the amount of time spent 'as player'. It is very easy, and indeed understandable, for such managers to give very high priority to their patients and clients and thus land up taking their management work

home at night. Planning 'chunks' of time when you are a player and chunks when you are a manager helps to overcome this dilemma. This pattern can be put in your diary, displayed on your wall planner and generally communicated to your colleagues so that you make it clear which of the two roles you are focusing on at any given time.

Identifying the time bandits and eliminating them

'The trick to saving time in your job is to work better not harder!' When faced with very long lists of activities, managers sometimes think that by working harder and for longer hours they will achieve more. While this is true to some extent, it is also true to say that if we used the time effectively and in particular identified and eliminated those things which 'steal' our time, we would be able to get through the list within the time planned.

Some typical time bandits and what to do about them

Paper work

Try to handle each piece of paper only once. Get into the habit of reading memos and letters with a pencil in your hand and, where at all possible, take immediate action. For example, write the answer on the memo and send it back, file it, send it on to the person who can deal with it or throw it away.

If possible, learn to write letters and memos on a dictating machine or input directly on to a personal computer if that is your way of working. If you have a secretary, run through the correspondence with the secretary, indicating the actions required.

If you do write memos and letters, try to keep them short, factual and to the point. If possible use e-mail, telephone or fax rather than write a letter.

In many organizations, staff complain about the very large flow of paper. For example, reports are often photocopied and circulated widely almost regardless of the relevance of the report to the individuals who receive them. As we mention in Chapter 8 on managing communication, a way to avoid wasting other people's time is to provide short (e.g. one side of an A4 piece of paper) summaries of long reports and to circulate the summary widely, indicating where the main report can be obtained. This helps to reduce the amount of reading time for individuals, but still allows them to determine whether the report is relevant to their work.

Telephone calls

Try to make your telephone calls in blocks. By doing this, you become more efficient in your handling of the calls and also if the first person you phone is not available, then you can deal with others and then try that person again later.

Have all the information you need to make your calls at hand on your desk. Spend a few seconds thinking about why you are calling someone; often making brief notes like an agenda is also helpful.

If your telephone calls come through a secretary or switchboard operator, ask that person to screen them for you or, if you need a quiet period of time to concentrate on some important piece of work, ask them to take names so that you can get back to them later. Use an answering machine as a way of filtering the calls and avoiding interruption. There is nothing more time-wasting in a meeting, for example, than a member constantly taking a few minutes to answer the telephone.

For people you telephone regularly, find out when is the best time for both of you to have a telephone conversation. This way you reduce the well-known cycle of 'I phone you and you are out, you phone back and I am out!'

Meetings (see also Chapter 6)

Always prepare an agenda or be aware of it when involved in meetings. Even informal meetings of small numbers can be made more effective by spending a few minutes in the beginning identifying what needs to be covered and how much time is available.

As well as having a start time for the meeting, agree a finish time. Whether you are chairing the meeting or attending it as a member, it is extremely valuable to know what the time scale is as you can then influence the amount of time spent on each item required to be covered.

Carry out a meeting audit. Look back over your diary say for the last month and calculate the number of meetings you attended and how much time was spent. Are you the right person to attend that meeting? Do you know why you are there? If you are the one who calls the meeting, was the use of the meeting the most effective way to deal with the work requiring to be undertaken? Managers spend a lot of time in meetings and it is worth being very critical of how that time is being spent and being quite ruthless in attendance, frequency and use of meetings.

Avoid the danger of meetings becoming cosy, social activities (unless of course that is what they are for, e.g. teambuilding). One company has installed a high table in their meeting room and removed the chairs. This has the effect of keeping meetings short and to the point!

Visitors

Work out who needs access to you at all times – e.g. your secretary if you have one, your senior managers and perhaps one or two other key members of staff – and clearly make yourself available to these people at all times. With other staff and external visitors, try to set up blocks of time when you are available, thus indicating when you do not wish to be disturbed.

When visitors come into your office, ask them politely how you can help them. It may also be useful to stand up when they come in. This signals to the visitor that, until you have determined the agenda, you will not invite them to sit down and take time to deal with the issue.

Visitors have come to see you because they want your help, advice or are seeking your permission. The phrase 'Have you got a minute?' is often the trigger for a lengthy and unplanned interruption. The skill lies in negotiating assertively with the visitor. Thus if you are very busy on important work, you can indicate that if it is a query that can be dealt with quickly then indeed you have got a minute. If it is important and needs more time, then perhaps a meeting should be scheduled for a longer period later in the day or the next day. Another technique is to block some time each week when you are available for visitors and publish this, thus also indicating when you are less available.

Case study 3.4

> Bill runs a social work section with five staff. He likes to think of himself as an 'open-door manager' and indeed is very good in his handling of staff problems and issues, providing good support and guidance. Staff come to discuss clients with him on a regular basis and he likes to keep in touch with what is going on. Unfortunately this approach has led to his day being filled with unplanned and *ad hoc* meetings – leaving him to take work home at night. He recognizes the need to be available to staff but longer term work is getting put back and then rushed.
>
> To take more control of the situation he plans the week to make chunks of time available for staff consultation and to reserve other time for his longer term work. He explains his problem to the staff at a meeting and gains their co-operation. They like this new system because they know when he can give full attention to their needs and also when he is not available, thus helping their use of time.

Managing your staff's time

The focus of this chapter so far has been on looking at the management of your own time. It follows that the principles and practices discussed apply equally to your staff. A number of specific practical points are worth outlining.

- Encourage your staff to establish a base line in relation to how they currently spend their time. This entails developing an appropriate time log so that they become aware of how time is spent. It is important to emphasize that the purpose of the time log is to help to identify ways to improve time management and is not about you 'checking up' on what each member of staff is doing. Use a team meeting to exchange experiences. The manager may be very surprised to find that typical time-wasters involve such things as the way the office is organized, difficulties in getting hold of each other, filing systems or even your approach as a boss. Whatever they are, you are more able now to find ways of improving the situation.

- Goal setting. Are your staff clear about their goals? Do you sit down, discuss and clarify goals from time to time? As has been stressed earlier in this chapter, the setting of goals helps to determine the ways in which time should be spent. If you are in any doubt at all about whether your staff fully understand their goals and how they fit into the work of the whole department, then you need to give this some urgent attention. If you have a career review or performance management scheme, this provides a regular mechanism for reviewing and agreeing goals.

- Staff often find difficulties in determining priorities of work. They may need your support in developing mechanisms for deciding upon priorities and particularly you may need to be available, if you are not already the source, to decide changes in priorities.

- Involving your staff in the planning process, particularly in terms of business plans for example, helps clarify how time can be deployed to meet the purpose of the department. The important issue here is to involve those who clearly are going to be central in meeting the goals in the setting of them. Your staff will know the detailed problems that are likely to be encountered and a great deal of time will be saved later if these problems are identified and handled at the planning stage.

- In more detailed terms, your staff might appreciate help in planning day-to-day work through encouragement of the use of daily lists, planners, etc. which may involve the provision of some resources, e.g. diaries and wall planners.

- Help your staff to identify the time-wasters (bearing in mind that you might be one of them!) and help to eliminate them. The use of the time logs will help to identify the major time-wasters; for example, are staff meetings being used as effectively as they might? It is particularly important to enable your staff to deal with time-wasters when in practice the solution to some of their problems may lie beyond their ability to solve them.

- Finally, try to stay open to suggestions from your staff about ways in which individually and collectively you can make more effective use of time. By creating a climate with your staff in which you are genuinely interested in seeking to improve time use you will increase the probability of good workable ideas coming forward.

Stress

So far in this chapter we have been looking at ways of improving management of time. It is important to look at the issue of stress as managers often report that they are experiencing stress and are looking for ways of managing it more effectively. This section explores the nature of stress, identifies some of the main sources and suggests some techniques for dealing with it.

In general terms, managing effectively can be a very demanding activity both physically and emotionally. Alongside this, we are often dealing with rapid change and we are expected to cope with all sorts of demands which can appear to be coming from several different directions at once. In this context, it is not surprising that people feel stressed.

Stress is experienced in a situation where you are forced to adapt or change in order to cope with something new. The 'challenges' that are faced in the public sector can represent problems which need to be solved. If, on the other hand, you have difficulty in solving these problems, the result can be stress. Thus challenges can be stressors if there is a mismatch between the demand and how you think you can deal with it, or you do not have the power to solve the problem as you would like, or you are lacking skills, sources or help or advice.

We know that different people are affected by stress in different ways and to different extents. In this sense what is a stressor for you, may not necessarily be a stressor for your boss or colleague. Stressors are very individual; this is probably the one key factor in helping us to understand and subsequently to deal with sources of stress. In order to deal with our stress we must first identify sources of stress for ourselves.

Some typical stressors are:

- Role ambiguity and lack of clear goals
- Lack of appropriate skills to cope with the change
- A feeling of lack of power or influence
- Over-demanding time deadlines
- Conflicts between personal and organizational values
- Personal relationships at work
- Too much (overload) or too little (underload) work
- Overly fast rate of change without time to evaluate the impact.

Activity

Take a moment to reflect on the sources of stress in work for you. Remember that stress is known for its impact on physical health but it can also affect the way you feel, think, react and behave. Certainly stress at work can affect your whole life because you may not be able to escape the pressures and tensions when you go home at night.

Positive aspects of stress

Some stress is good for you! We probably need some stress to provide the push to get us to start acting in order to achieve some goals. This stress acts as a form of motivation, making you feel slightly anxious and worried about getting some things done. Provided that it is at a relatively manageable level, this is experienced as 'rust-out', i.e. it gets you going. The problem is when the number and levels of stressors cause you to approach 'burn-out' when no amount of longer hours or working harder seems to improve the situation.

So, if you have a better idea now of your sources of stress, what can you do about them? Essentially you have two options: you can seek to avoid the sources of stress or you can develop coping mechanisms for dealing with them.

Avoiding strategies

These include using the time management advice we have outlined above, that is to try to anticipate, plan and avoid situations which overload you with stress. In the more extreme form, if work is making you really unhappy then perhaps you need to review your career, how it fits in with your personal life and ask yourself whether some change of organization or direction in your life is the real solution.

Coping mechanisms

These involve a range of techniques aimed at trying to help you deal with day-to-day pressures and stress in situations where the source of stress cannot be avoided. Consider the following strategies.

- Always express your feelings about pressures at work – talk to your boss, your colleagues or your partner, but above all communicate about it. The process of sharing your perception about the pressures you are experiencing to a sympathetic listener helps to put that situation in perspective and help and advice (and hopefully understanding) coming from one of these sources will support you at a stressful time.
- Try to take a broad view of your work situation every so often – the 'helicopter vision' we referred to on page 22. As someone eloquently put it: *'When you are up to your eyes in the swamp and the alligators are snapping at your heels it's difficult to remember that the reason you are in the swamp in the first place was to drain it and get rid of the alligators!'*
  If you have a clear picture of your longer term goals, the shorter term fire-fighting becomes more manageable; you can also spend some time trying to improve the overall situation so that you have fewer alligators to deal with.
- Alter your perception. Try to see a stressful situation as an opportunity for you to develop new skills, new techniques and grow. In any challenging situation try to take time occasionally *to reflect* on what you have

learnt from that situation: for example, how would you manage a similar situation in the future or how would you plan to avoid it? This positive thinking approach is clearly difficult when you are in the stressful setting but with practice it is possible to get better.

● Examine the time balance in your life:

Activity

Essentially, we spend our time in one of three ways:

● work activity;
● support activities, e.g. sleeping, eating, carrying out chores of various kinds; and
● relaxation and leisure, e.g. being with friends and family, sports, hobbies, interests, etc.

Think of a typical week (168 hours). Calculate how many hours you spend in each of the areas:

Work	hours	Percentage =		%
Support	hours	Percentage =		%
Relaxation	hours	Percentage =		%
Total		(168 hours)	100%	

We need to ensure that we have a balance between work, support and relaxation activities: perhaps 25–35 per cent on *work* activity, 45–55 per cent in *support* and 15–25% in *relaxation*. How did your time balance compare to this? What do you want to achieve?

If work is making too many demands on us the first casualty is usually our relaxation time. While this is acceptable for short periods, if it has become the norm then we have to try to ensure that we give ourselves time for relaxation, which in turn will improve our performance in work.

● Try to develop a habit of taking some exercise and relaxation on a regular basis, e.g. 10–15 minutes a day. This does not have to be vigorous exercise, it can be as simple as taking a walk or doing a few stretching exercises, for instance, of a yoga type. The main point is that you are trying to keep fit and giving yourself a change from the work situation. Try walking upstairs instead of taking the lift, walking to work occasionally or taking a swim before work in the morning or at lunchtime. The important points are that the form of exercise suits you and that you develop a habit of ensuring you get some time to yourself.

These are a small number of suggestions that you can try out as appropriate; no doubt you will have already developed some coping strategies but we hope that this list has added to your range.

The main message of this section is that you must try to take control of stressful situations rather than to let them appear to take control of you. The ability to negotiate and the development of assertiveness will also prove useful strategies in dealing with stress and these are discussed elsewhere in the book.

Conclusion

Time management starts with your desire to make more effective use of your time at work. Without this motivation to take control, making progress is difficult. It is all too easy to point to the 'system' or other people and say that 'they take up all your time'.

This chapter has attempted to outline the principles of effective time and stress management and explored many practical ways to proceed which value and respect others but recognize your needs too.

Further reading

Atkinson P E (1988) *Achieving Results through Time Management*. Pitman, London.

Fleming I (1990) *The Time Management Pocketbook*. Management Pocketbooks, Alresford.

Holden R (1992) *Stress Busters. Over 101 Strategies for Stress Survival*. Thorsons, London.

Mackay I and Gill D (1990) *A Guide to Managing Time*. BACIE 1990, London.

Noon J A (1990) *Time – The Busy Manager's Action Plan for Effective Self Management*. Chapman & Hall, London.

4

The manager as communicator

In this chapter we deal with communication as a joint responsibility between speaker and listener, sender and receiver; aspects of listening and negotiation; some of the key issues in interviewing and presentation, together with an overview of transactional analysis as a technique for appreciating the tone and manner of our communication.

Communication skills and processes

'Well', says the senior to his staff, 'they were told, so they should have known!' Many people share this view of communication and see it solely as the 'telling' part of the exercise. (Some view communication as: 'tell them and then tell them again – louder!'). This is a very common opinion, it implies, 'I've done the job, passed the message – over and OUT' Is this successful communication?

Successful communication is a *sharing process:* a partnership between the sender and receiver with both having some responsibility for the success of the communication.

Feedback and communication

Have you ever played a game where you sit back to back with a partner and he or she has to explain a drawing or shape to you? In one variant of this game you, the receiver, are not allowed to say anything; you have merely to listen hard to what you are being told. The results of this partnership are usually poor: the two drawings hardly correspond. You then might have tried this exercise with the receiver being allowed to ask questions as he or she is being informed of the task. The results are usually better: the drawing does sometimes resemble the original. This suggests that where there is feedback from the receiver to the sender then generally the accuracy of communication will be greater. This feedback occurs when the questions are asked, the attempts at clarification and expansion provided. ('Did you say the base of the triangle was 3 cm to the right, or was it the left ?') All this may not matter much when we are simply playing a game involving drawings, but it can and often does make a crucial difference when instructions are passed in a health or social care setting.

Without feedback, it is like operating in the dark

Where there is no feedback then the sender is often operating in the dark having to make assumptions as to whether the communication has been successfully received and understood or not. This 'darkness' can be rendered a little less dense if the sender knows something about the person or persons being communicated with, about their likely perceptions, attitudes and expectations. If we are just 'shooting into the dark' then we have to be very careful about any assumptions we may make; such a reliance can sometimes have unexpected and alarming results.

A dramatic example of this occurred some years ago in the Clapham rail disaster. A message distribution system failed to work because staff who needed to see the new safety regulations for testing signals were not required to acknowledge receipt of them; the reason given at the Court of Inquiry was 'to save administrative effort'. The supervisor had 'assumed' the new rules had been received by everyone and were being implemented. This assumption was not long in being tested: the train hurtled through the wrong signals with fatal results for many of the passengers. It does not take too much effort to translate this scenario into a care setting. 'I had assumed the theatre sister had been told of the new procedures' or 'but I thought that following my memo, procedures were now in place in the community'.

Testing our assumptions about communication

More recently there was a case written up in the Sunday newspapers of a Trust executive who had placed himself in a wheelchair outside the casualty department of one of his hospitals with a supposed lack of feeling in his legs and some pain. He told in the article of how one by one his assumptions concerning customer service standards and agreed working procedures that he had believed were being kept by staff were in fact not being implemented and that procedures very different from those stipulated were in fact the order of the day. Putting to one side the ethics of this bit of research, what would you find as a manager if you went into one of your units, sections or departments? Would your assumptions of what your staff were doing stand up to such scrutiny?

Activity

Consider this whole aspect of making assumptions about the.way communications are being received and understood. Have you been able to set up systems which enable you to test out such assumptions: to monitor communication success or failure? If not, how would you avoid this Clapham Effect?

Responsibilities for successful communication

From what we have said so far it appears as though the sender has most of the responsibility for the communication. One can argue that if the message (defined in the broadest sense) is sent in such a way so as to allow those that receive it to be able to easily understand it (i.e. it is put into accessible language, it is not too long and involved) then some part of the responsibility for communication does lie with the receiver. When the channel tunnel was being constructed and French and English workers were working side by side, the rule at Eurotunnel was that, first, speakers had to make sure they said what they were supposed to by way of an instruction or request, and secondly, it was the listener's responsibility to understand. The rule said clearly: 'If you don't understand, you've got to bloody well say so!' Likewise at Gatwick Airport there is a series of prominent signs which state: 'There are no announcements in this airport, passengers should check the screens for information on departures and arrivals.' In other words, the responsibility for getting to the right plane at the right time is yours.

Who do we blame? Speaker or listener?

This is not a fashionable or easy line to take: we all tend to blame the sender and not think that we as listeners have a responsibility. 'It was the doctor's fault I didn't understand the dosage; the guard's fault that we got on to the wrong platform and definitely that fellow's fault that we got on to the wrong road after we stopped and asked him – he got us into a right old muddle with all that carry on about third left after the second roundabout.'

Activity

Consider the question: Do your staff think you should take the responsibility for communicating?

All these examples illustrate the crucial importance of checking details, asking questions, making sense of the communication for ourselves. Yeats the Irish poet once said: 'Somewhere between my reading of the poem and the audience's listening to the poem, the poem is'. We could say that somewhere between the teller who is taking care to make the message accessible and the listener who is keeping alert and checking out the information – communication is!

The problem in so much of health and social care is that staff, patients and clients do not ask questions or check details enough. They do not in fact take much responsibility for sharing the communication.

Activity

Why do you think it is often so difficult for these groups to share this responsibility? Think carefully of your own situation before you read on. How do you check on information? How do you try to encourage your staff to take on more of this responsibility?

We wonder if you would agree that the following factors are to blame.

- A traditional view of inter-staff and staff/patient relationships which encourages staff, patients and clients to believe that it is their place to be told and not to question.
- A management/leadership style that pays only lip service to communication as a sharing process as opposed to direction of staff, patients and clients.
- Poor procedures in terms of communication to staff: slipshod briefings, unclear notices and memos.
- Failure of management to 'sell' the importance of communication to staff; to assist and train staff in communication skills; to point out the responsibilities of listening by checking and verifying information before passing it on.
- A lack of awareness of the importance of communication and its central place in the workplace.

Are there others you feel we have missed that you are aware of in your workplace?

Attitudes and expectations affect communications

There is ample evidence as to the effects of attitudes on the way we both send and receive communication. A report by the Audit Commission, *Trusting in the Future* (1993), identified staff apathy, resistance to change, fear, uncertainty and cynicism as being prevalent within many NHS hospitals. With such a climate it is no surprise that attitudes can have a marked effect on the way in which communication from management is received. On a more personal level if we have a negative attitude to the person we are communicating with then this may well affect the way in which we send our message. Consider the example in Case study 4.1.

Case study 4.1

> The senior nurse considers the student nurse to be rather slow – she has heard this opinion from others on the ward – so she does not bother giving her a very full explanation. Because of this the student cannot think of any points on which to question her. This lack of stimulation reinforces the negative attitude held by the senior nurse; this shows itself in passive communication, and leads towards the self-fulfilling prophecy: 'Well I'm glad I didn't waste much time giving her a detailed account'.

If we as managers are to succeed in communicating with our colleagues, staff, patients and clients then we have to take attitudes into consideration. So often 'improvements' in communication are made at a mechanical level: 'Let's have a new noticeboard?' 'We ought to make our memos more readable'. 'How about launching a team briefing system?' These aspects are obviously important but if staff attitudes are not taken into consideration then there may well be a neutral effect at best or negative one at worst and much money and managers' time may be wasted.

We have come across examples of team briefings (systems designed to get information through an organization as quickly as possible via meetings to cascade the 'brief' down from management to all staff) that have been instituted but that appear to have petered out because of some staff resistance and lack of enthusiasm on the part of middle managers. Clearly communication of the wrong or inappropriate kind can do more harm than good; it can lead to a loss of credibility in the source and can make it that much harder to launch a new communication initiative. Of course it is a manager's job to lead, to go out front and provide a vision, but it is also important to make sure that the others are following and have been told where you are heading. We should therefore keep the *staff's attitudes and expectations* firmly in mind when we plan, structure and send / present our communication. Let us look at each of these stages in more detail.

Plan

Having asked ourselves the most obvious of questions: do we actually need this piece of communication and is there an alternative? we then ask: who is the audience? Is this broadcast, i.e. to be sent to a large number of staff/ patients and clients? or is it narrowcast – directed at a small, specialized group who will be familiar with specialized terms (such as narrowcast!)? A crucial question to ask is: what is my audience likely to think of this material, will they see it as important, useful or relevant? What are their likely expectations? Has there been a communication similar to this in the recent past and can this be built on to it in some way? Is there any method by which

I can show its importance, usefulness or relevance, perhaps with an example (selected with suitable care), with a case study drawn from recent experience, with a call for action, an invitation to respond via way of information gathering, etc.? How can I demonstrate the urgency of this communication?

Most texts on presentation skills lay stress on the need to prepare the material to be delivered. But crucially it is the consideration of the audience's likely *attitudes* to the material that is often the most important part of this preparation. If we simply blast our way through this attitudinal wall then we know that many of our listeners will select out, distort, rubbish and discount what we say. We have learnt enough from health education campaigns, for example, to realize that to break through the attitudinal barrier we must counter argument with argument, case with case, appreciate the likely (and to our minds perhaps unwise) *rationalizations* our audience will have on our subject and be prepared to use subtle persuasive measures to win a hearing.

Structure

It is important to organize any material into a structure which can be readily understood. How can I gain the attention of my readers – hook their attention? You might consider this pattern:

- What is this communication about? Why should I read it or listen to it?
- What do I need to do as a result of my reading/listening to it? Consider the language level (*separate* for discrete, *match* for commensurate), the use of jargon, e.g., empowerment.

Sending

When and how should it be sent? In one issue or in episodes? Should it be sent in full or would a summary be enough? Should it be sent to each member of the audience or to a representative for it to be sent along channels? In what form should it be sent: orally, on paper, by e-mail, as a notice, as an article within the staff magazine/bulletin?

There is also a fourth, very important stage which is often left out of the process.

The follow-up

Most communication has a very short shelf life; it decays rapidly. People quickly forget and the pressure of immediate business often drives your memo from their minds. This is why it is important to plan for some kind of follow-up, and without too much delay. This may be in the form of a simple reminder letter or memo, a series of phone calls, a meeting or a sandwich lunch with a key group of staff. Failure to follow up a communication runs the risk of it not being taken seriously or of it decaying slowly. A follow-up also invites the receivers to take some responsibility for the success of the communication, to develop some degree of ownership in the outcomes. It also allows you another attempt to pierce the attitudinal walls which may have been thrown up at your first presentation or delivery; very often we are not persuaded on first acquaintance; it takes time for us to warm to the sender and his or her message.

Activity

Read the account given in Case study 4.2 and consider what advice you would give to the various parties represented.

Case study 4.2

The personnel director is keen to communicate to all staff the new arrangements for contracts. He brings it up at a Board of Management meeting where it is discussed briefly. Members agree that this is a crucial item and deserves a meeting to itself. The personnel director informally gives some information to a senior officer who passes it on at her next staff meeting. Meanwhile a week later the Board of Management address the issue of contracts at their meeting, agree a policy and ask this to be communicated to all staff as soon as possible. The personnel director takes this duty on as his responsibility.

He issues a memo to be sent to each staff member but decides to wait 10 days so that it can be included in the wage/salary slips. He writes as follows:

Dear Staff Member
As some of you may be aware, the Board of Management has decided at its meeting on 19th December to go ahead with the issue of new contracts for staff. Your departmental/sector managers and supervisors will be communicating the details to you.

A series of meetings is held between the director of personnel and managers and supervisors, the purpose being to fully brief them so that they are able to explain the changes in detail to their staff groups. Unfortunately, because of the Christmas and New Year holidays several delays creep into their sequencing. At these meetings it is obvious that some managers have already found out about these changes – some have heard of them via their staff, others through the grapevine. There is some ill feeling amongst these managers and complaints are voiced to the director of personnel as to the manner in which the information was 'leaked'.

The briefing continues and the changes are explained via the use of overhead projectors and handouts. Information packs to be given out to each member of staff are also distributed. The director of personnel sets aside time to answer particular questions during the session and also announces the times and dates that he is available for consultation/advice from any manager/supervisor who needs help over any issue with their particular staff members. He receives some questions at the meeting but no one takes up his offer of consultation. There appears to be some bewilderment!

At the next Board of Management meeting on 11 January there is considerable disquiet expressed by members of the lack of consistency in the way that managers had explained the new contracts to their respective staff groups. The director of personnel was asked to send out a detailed memo to correct what members felt had been a wrong interpretation given by some managers, particularly with regard to part-time staff.

The memo is sent out, it begins:

> Dear Staff Member
> With reference to memo sent to staff on Dec 20th with regard to new contracts, the Board of Management has asked me to clarify several points:

It then goes on to list these. During that day and the next the director of personnel's office is kept very busy dealing with phone calls. These are from managers feeling aggrieved that their briefings have appeared to be criticized and from individual members of staff, particularly part-timers, requesting further clarification as where they now stand with regard to the new contracts. The organizers of the various trades unions and professional groups are also actively seeking interviews with the director.

Discussion of Case study 4.2

Planning

You could safely say, 'not a lot'. There was far too little thought given to how this very important, even crucial, information was to be passed to staff – both full and part-timers. There were various stages in this communication and it appears that there was not enough detailed planning of each stage and the likely difficulties that might be encountered. With such important information, consultation with trade unions and professional associations should have been planned for at the very start. You might also consider it unwise to launch such a major initiative over the Christmas and New Year period.

Channels of communication

Although it is a very good practice to make use of a variety of channels when communicating a message (think how the advertisers do it with posters, TV advertising, product displays in supermarkets, etc.), we should be careful to limit ourselves to one main channel to avoid the danger, as happened here, of information leaking out in advance of the main announcement. You may have experienced the results of this kind of thing: some staff appear to know more than others, the rumour mill becomes very active and many people get disgruntled, irritated or even more cynical about all information reaching them from management. You might also consider it unwise to allow a period of 10 days to elapse before sending out the information in the wage/salary slips. You might also question the wisdom of sending out such information through that route.

Vagueness

The memos written by the personnel director are magnificent specimens of the art of vagueness. These are the sort of memos that inspire disquiet in the mind of the reader – what has been left out? Why, 'as some of you may be aware'? – that is rather a worrying statement, implying some are more favoured than others in the communication stakes. We should note that in any situation where there is unequal access to communication, jealousies and suspicions may be aroused.

Failure to listen

We must admit that there was a distinct failure by the Board of Management to focus properly on the words of their personnel director when he first outlined his plan to them. Responsibilities for subsequent failures should lie at their door. Attentive listening should have brought out questions, calls for clarification, amplification and elaboration.

You may have been reminded of the game of Chinese whispers reading this case study. You remember from that game the alarming way in which even a simple message is distorted and elaborated by the very fact of its being passed from person to person. You can imagine with this health board scenario the effects of rumour and distortion. Where there are likely to be negative attitudes to a communication then this distortion will be even greater. People will tend to distort a message to bring it into line with their own attitudes and prejudices.

The director of personnel did well to get the group together in an attempt to brief them. However after a briefing on such an important matter it is surprising that there were no questions. Perhaps his listeners were too stunned, shocked by the news? Perhaps it had come as a great surprise to them. It may have been that they were overawed in his presence and clammed up. Perhaps he had made the assumption that since the briefing was comprehensive, there would be no need to question it. We can probably say again with some confidence that members of that group did bear some of the responsibility for subsequent failure by not asking questions, by not verifying the information. Let us leave the case study for the moment and turn to some specific skills of communication.

Some interpersonal skills

Listening

How much time do you as a manager spend listening (or trying to do so) to your staff, colleagues, patients and clients? Several surveys of managers' time allocation suggest that over a third of the working week is spent in some kind of listening activity, either in interviews, at meetings, on the telephone or from tapes on answering machines. How would you score in such a survey? You may not spend a third of your time listening but we are certain it will be a very significant proportion of your time. It is curious that although much of managing others is spent in listening, little training occurs to improve the quality of this process.

Activity

What do you think makes for a good listener? Try writing out your own list of the qualities you consider important before you continue reading.

Here is our checklist. A good listener:

- does his or her best to fight off attitudes/prejudice and stereotypes of the speaker, and listens to the words rather than the person saying them and judges content not speaker;
- fights against being switched off by any interference, noise, distracting habits of the speaker (which we may be causing);
- waits until he or she has understood the key ideas before jumping in;
- provides limited but encouraging response to the speaker – enough to keep the channel open but not so much that it appears the listener is taking over;
- fights against switching off when confronted by a very slow/hesitant speaker, and counteracts by anticipating/summarizing what is said; and
- takes the odd note, records key words, ideas, figures.

Did you have many more?

Listening and negotiation

Listening is very much linked to negotiation and assertive behaviours. If we are feeling under pressure and not happy that we have allowed ourselves to be put into a position where we feel stuck with someone, then we will be unlikely to be able to listen carefully and in accordance with the principles listed above. Very often unless we secure a space for ourselves by being assertive or through negotiation then we will be looking over our shoulders, at the clock, planning our journey and just not attending. One hallmark of a good listener is the ability after the speaker has finished to provide a summary of the key points. This is a difficult task to do unless the listener is concentrating carefully.

The first part of the negotiation in any situation where one is actively listening is to clarify exactly what is the aim and the agenda. So often we are trying to find out answers to: What is this all about? Does it concern me? Where will it lead?, that we are not really paying much attention. Once we have clarified the aim and agenda, we can focus our concentration on the task at hand by questioning, clarifying, summarizing, paraphrasing, etc.

Effective listening tends to take place when the listener has sufficient confidence to negotiate the terms under which any listening occurs. Furthermore, according to some research (Anderson et al., 1985), when faced with incoming information that is confused, incoherent or not consistent, the effective listener does something about it such as asking and clarifying. The research indicated that increased confidence and promptness in clarifying the issue enabled much better communication to develop.

This adds further weight to the need for responsible listening. Taking notes may be helpful here: the very process of jotting down key words and ideas may assist us in tuning in to what is being said. However, care has to be taken not to put the speaker off by scribbling notes and not managing to stay within eye contact. We have to be careful, therefore, that in taking notes we do not interrupt the flow of communication, annoy the speaker or cause alarm by allowing him or her to worry about the confidentiality of the notes being taken. Two tips: always leave plenty of space in your notes for future amplification, i.e. leave wide margins, and do not forget to write up any notes as soon as possible after the interview.

Interviewing

There is no way in this text that we can cover the whole of interviewing – selection, appraisal, disciplinary, etc. We refer you to excellent texts that do. What we would like to do is survey some principal communication skills, including listening, that managers need as interviewers. We develop many of these points when we examine appraisal interviewing in Chapter 14.

All interviews depend for their success on *preparation:* of the situation, the paper work, the questions to be asked, the follow-up, etc. We are sure that many of you reading this will have experienced being interviewed and the feeling that the whole performance was rushed and badly prepared.

We can itemize this preparation:

- *Purpose of interview.* Is this clear to you and the interviewee? This is especially important in disciplinary and grievance interviews. Any uncertainty over role will have negative effects on performance.
- *Players.* Who is to take part? Have they been given plenty of warning and been adequately briefed? Are they the most appropriate players in terms of skills, experience, interest, etc.? (By the way what are you as manager doing about training, coaching and encouraging interview skills amongst your subordinates and colleagues?)
- *Paper work.* Are you confident that all the players, including the interviewees, are getting the paper they need at the right time and in the most readable format for them to perform at their best during the interview: application forms, appraisal reports, references, etc.?
- *Procedures.* Have you checked with your staff that such aspects as reception areas, the payment of expenses, etc., is organized?
- *Environment.* Have you had a really good look at the room/s in which the interview/s will take place? Have you put yourself in the chair that the interviewee will sit in and considered the view that he or she will have of you? Where is that desk lamp shining? Will it appear to be more of an interrogation than a constructive discussion?
- *Review* It is very important that any interviewing procedure should be reviewed on occasions. As part of such a review the opinions of those interviewed should be sought as well as those who carry out the interviews. It is all too easy for an interviewing process to 'get stuck' in some kind of organizational rut. It is often useful to view the interview procedures of other, similar organizations to yours as well as other health and social care services in order to see how they manage things.

This is a form of 'benchmarking' and is related to the way in which we set standards. It implies that there is always someone out there who can do it better. It relates to our discussion on quality in Chapter 12. Now let us take a brief look at two of the main interviews that feature in management.

Selection interviews

Many interviewers have a very optimistic view of their abilities in picking winners. Research (Statt, 1994) does not present such a rosy picture. In 20–40 minutes (the normal duration) what can we do? Can we really estimate intelligence, moral courage, honesty, ability to work under pressure, communication skills and...? Goodworth (1985) suggests that the whole purpose of any selection interview is 'to carry out a comprehensive and accurate background investigation to seek out and verify the facts of past achievement'. If we follow his line of argument then as selectors we must pay very close attention to what the CV says, what aspects have been highlighted in the application and how all this measures up to the job description.

There is much to be said for the line of reasoning that the best indicator of a person's performance is his or her previous record of achievement. As one speaker at a recent Institute of Personnel Management conference said, 'If you want to find a good team leader, ask his or her present team their opinion of his or her leadership, don't just accept what is said or written by the referees'. Hence we should very carefully *read and check* the information we have on the applicants and how these apply to the job description we have outlined. We have seen the effects of attitudes on our listening. In the interview we have to be especially careful that we do not close out the incoming information by sieving it through our prejudices and hearing only what we want or expect to hear. Likewise we have to watch out for the well-known 'halo effect', so-called because one positive or negative attribute helps shape our opinion of the candidate. We are all susceptible to such halos and to the effect of them on our judgements of people.

Questioning

We have to verify, clarify and seek amplification of these 'key facts of past achievement' as Goodworth (1985) puts them and to do this we have to use a variety of questions and not rely on simple closed questions which invite the answer yes or no and the open which provide plenty of scope for the candidate to expand: 'How did you feel about...?' We should make full use of the clarification questions: 'Could you explain a little more...?' or 'Could you give us an example...?'

Let us face it, if we do not ask we don't get. Those at interview are unlikely to volunteer damaging information about themselves. Have you ever?

Appraisal interviews

We deal with appraisal in Chapter 14. The aim is to review a person's employment, his or her achievements and strengths and those areas where support and training need to be given – the shortfall. As with all interviewing, effective and thorough preparation is the key. The appraiser should have read the appraisee's job description, background information relating to the post and be updated on performance standards as reported by the supervisor or manager. The appraisee should know the purpose and scope of the interview, have had time to write up his or her view of the year's performance, the achievements and targets met and the areas where further effort was necessary.

The aim of the appraisal is to reach a level of joint agreement and a shared understanding between the two parties as to the outcome of the interview. The goal is to reach an agreed statement of aims and targets to be reached before the next appraisal. Promises and commitments arrived at during the interview must be clarified and there should be a written statement setting out the agreement; this should be signed by both parties.

Presentation

Another of the crucial skills for the manager is the ability to present information to colleagues in a clear, concise and well-structured manner. There are plenty of texts on this, and training videos. Here we outline some key stages.

First, as we have mentioned earlier in this chapter, we need to understand and appreciate the likely expectations and attitudes of our audiences. Let us take these in turn.

Expectations

So often a presentation goes wrong, the audience is left feeling disappointed and the speaker rather hurt because expectations have not matched up; the audience expected – were led to believe – that the manager would cover the whole of subject X whereas he or she had in fact just outlined his or her own views on the subject. Our advice is to check and double check with the person who invites you to make the presentation just what exactly are the 'terms of reference'. You may well have to negotiate these: the expectations of the audience may not be realizable within the time that you have either for the preparation of the material or for the duration of the talk itself.

Attitudes

We all listen through a filter of our attitudes and stereotypes. We have already said that in carrying out interviews it is very important to actually listen to what is being said and do your best to filter out your own attitudes. When you are preparing the subject matter for your presentation do consider the likely objections, rationalizations of your listeners. These rationalizations may not be 'correct' or even very scientific as far as you are concerned but they are the audience's. If they are likely to be holding negative views to yours then you will need to acknowledge these and provide reasons, examples, illustrations to back up your position. It is very important that your own commitment and enthusiasm for your views comes across.

Enthusiasm

In order to appear enthusiastic it is vital that the presentation should not be read line by line from a page but delivered with maximum eye contact with your audience. Even if you have to deliver a conference paper, do aim to look up from the prepared text as much as possible. The more negative the audience are to you and your proposals or information, the more the need to look at them – not stare – but keep contact with all of them. So do make sure you are very well prepared and that you know what you want to say so that you can use any notes that you have very much as cues which will allow you to maintain this contact. Remember also that we gather that someone is enthusiastic by the way something is said – the way that key points are stressed. It is no good saying something's 'vital' if it is said with lowered voice and a dull vocal tune – the audience will not be very convinced that it is so vital.

Structure

It is very important in any presentation to structure it so that the introduction – the reason why you are speaking – is clear to your listeners; that the main points are obvious (3 or 4, not many more); and that they know when you have reached the conclusion. For many presentations consider using PREP:

- P – State your position – why you are taking up their time
- R – Provide a reason – state the key points
- E – Give an example – it always helps make a general point clear
- P – Restate your position by way of a conclusion.

This is similar to one of the oldest and best pieces of advice in the business: 'Say what you are going to say, say it and then say what you've said.'

Visual appeal

Remember that you are the main attraction, people have come to hear you and not to see twenty overhead slides. Any such slides, flip chart sheets, etc. must be regarded as a complement to you and what you say. There is no doubt that a simple visual aid well prepared and carefully slotted into a talk can considerably enhance a presentation. However, you have probably had to sit through talks during which the speaker's attention has become mesmerized by some hand-written slide, the contents of which could not be read, and just as you managed to decipher them the slide was withdrawn, leaving you none the wiser. A baffled and irritated audience is not one to recommend. Keep all visuals simple, clear in layout (no more than six lines of absolutely no more than six words in 14 point type face bold) and do supply paper copies of each slide for your audience, and announce the fact before you speak so that your audience is not trying to make notes and so half hear what you are saying.

Questions

There is no good reason why questions should always and only be at the end of a presentation. In fact because of the general urgency of getting to coffee or a parking meter, it is a good idea to build in a definite break for questions at some convenient (that is convenient for yourself) point. Do remember that if you say to your audience, 'Stop me at any time if you'd like me to answer a question' then (a) you have to mean it and (b) you must know your material very well so that you will not be thrown off track as can easily happen.

Follow-up

Most of the real influencing at a presentation takes place at the follow-up via telephone, letter, fax, coffee or lunch meeting. No matter how brilliant your presentation, much of it will be quickly forgotten. That is why it is important to provide your listeners with a summary of the key points as a handout.

Nerves

Most people do not like giving presentations. One way of reducing the nervous tension is to consider that most audiences are on your side – meaning that they want your presentation to 'work'. When we are in an audience we dislike the embarrassment of a failure – a speaker drying up for instance. So if you stick to your remit, stick to your allotted time, look at the audience, avoid embarrassing or insulting them, make a few points in a well-structured manner then they will stay with you – they may not agree with your argument but they will respect your efforts.

Do try and start your presentation slowly: a flustered rapid start with nervous rearrangement of papers, rapid switching on and off of overhead projectors and a rapid machine-gun-like introduction can all have the effect of unsettling the audience. Your job is to settle them, so start slowly and do not start speaking until your audience have settled and are ready.

We hope this section has provided you with useful ideas for your presentations. In our next section we survey a framework which can be used for all your communication, be it a presentation, interview or telephone conversation, report, memo or fax.

Transactional analysis

There are many excellent texts on the market which cover this approach to interpersonal communications. What follows is a brief sketch which we hope will give you a starting point, or refresh your knowledge if you have come across Transactional Analysis (TA) before.

Think of your cassette player and a tape running around inside. The tape represents the various communications you habitually use (the transactions). You presumably seldom pick up a piece of tape to examine the magnetic coatings, and, apart from the occasional cleaning of the heads inside the tape player, you do not carry out much maintenance. TA suggests that because our communication with others is so habitual, so predictable and usual that it is a good idea to stop the 'tape' and have a serious look at what is being said and how it is being expressed. TA suggests that if we do not carry out a little maintenance of our communication systems they may become reduced in efficiency.

There is a great deal more to TA than this brief sketch allows; however, the essence is that all our communications with others can be improved and that we should become more sensitive to the transactions that we give off to others – for instance our staff, colleagues, patients and clients – and also become more sensitive to those transactions which we receive from others. Who is there on your staff who can tell you about the quality of your 'transactions'?

Briefly then there are three main 'states' as TA calls them, any one of which we may use when communicating. These are the 'adult', the 'parent' and the 'child'. The *adult* contains those aspects to do with objective rather than subjective behaviour, such as when we are analysing, testing and observing. This state is therefore one we use when interviewing: it creates the appropriate 'level' tone that is desirable. The *parent* contains the attitudes, feelings and behaviours associated with parental behaviours: laying down rules, criticizing and punishing. There is also the nurturing parent side which is about fostering, and helping – very important parts of the manager's role with staff. The *child* contains all the impulsive behaviours that come naturally to a child: joy, love, frustrations, tears and anger. It is a state full of very negative and also very positive emotions. What do you feel is your predominant 'state'? What reply would your staff and colleagues give?

TA suggests that we need to appreciate these various states in order that we can avoid becoming 'stuck' in any one of them and also so that we can appreciate the effects on our transactions with others if we operate from a particular state.

Stuck states

We have already suggested that managers will need to adopt the nurturing parent role. In Chapter 14 we take these ideas further when examining delegation and motivation. Staff will come with problems and will need to be supported and cared for. On the other hand staff will also come with good news, success stories and achievements to their credit. This is when the 'child' state needs to surface: joy breaks out, fun is had, handshakes (and hugs) distributed. So many managers seem to be unable to express joy and share in celebration; this can have a crippling effect on staff morale. For most of the time as managers we will need to adopt the adult state: being impartial, being objective, not letting our natural feelings rise too quickly to the surface. But we must be careful that this adult is not the only face that our staff see. Have you ever worked for such a manager? Did you enjoy the experience?

The second reason for becoming 'unstuck' in our states is that we can appreciate the effect of these on our communication. If we tend to address staff from the critical 'parent' state we should not be too surprised to find they react in the 'child' (Figure 4.1).

TA does not promise that if we address people from an adult state we will always get an adult reaction – far from it, there may be all kinds of deep attitudes and past transactions which contaminate our adult and cause us to snap back or sulk at a seemingly neutral adult question or statement. TA also

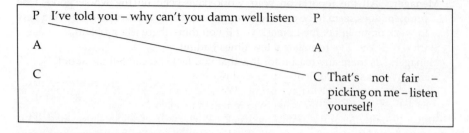

Figure 4.1 A 'parent' type remark will often elicit a 'child' type response.

suggests that it is not only the words used but the non verbal gestures and paralinguistic tones which create the transactions. Therefore we should be sensitive to how we use gestures – pointing at people for instance. Have a look at this extract from an appraisal interview to see how TA can help explain what happens.

> Manager:　Come in. Just sit there. I'll be with you in a moment (writes and makes phone call) You'll know what this is all about.... I've read all the reports on you by your supervisor. In general things appear OK. Would you agree?
> Staff:　Well, yes...
> Manager:　Fine. I'm not too happy by his comments on some of your time-keeping
> Staff:　Could I just say....
> Manager:　He notes that you've been late six times in the last month – that really won't do, will it ?
> Staff:　(stands up) I've had enough. (walks out and slams the door)

Activity

> We said earlier that it was crucial to create the appropriate tone in such an interview. Why has this gone so wrong? List your reasons before you continue reading.

Your list may contain:

- Critical parent opening shown by boss.
- No real welcome either in verbal or non-verbal approaches (head down writing notes suggests he cannot be bothered much; his making the phone call in her presence further marginalizes her).
- Rude interruptions over her comments; use of critical parent words such as: 'that really won't do'. No wonder her 'child' surfaced and she walked out.

The study of TA should help us recognize when we are using the critical parent and go very slow on it. A more adult approach would have enabled the manager to get at the problem of lateness. Compare:

Manager: All the reports on your work have been on the whole good. One problem does seem to be coming through and that is timekeeping – getting here to work on time. Let me first ask you if you think there is a problem.

Staff: Well yes, I've been late a few times I admit.

Manager: Is there any reason for this that you feel you can tell me about?

Staff: Well it's a bit difficult – personal reasons.

Manager: I don't have to have details. We need to make sure that this problem can be solved. Can I ask if it is likely to remain a problem?

Staff: I'm moving at the end of the week – I'm leaving...well let's just say that I'll be within a bus ride of work instead of being stuck out in the sticks having to rely on him bringing me in.

Manager: Would you like me to have a word with your supervisor on this?

Staff: No thanks, I don't think it'll be a problem after next week.

Manager: Fine. Could we now move on to...

You may well say that all that took a lot of time and the manager might simply have told her to stop coming in late or there would be trouble. Yes, and that approach can work, but would it have enabled the staff member to express her feelings, give her opinions and develop some 'ownership' in the proceedings? Many health and social care organizations proclaim ownership and empowerment of staff. We wonder how many interviews still present a parent-to-child aspect ? Berne, the founder of TA, said that it was not only individuals who could get stuck in their states but whole organizations could become parental, driving their staff into childish behaviours, such as deliberate lateness, making fake sickness claims, defacing memos on walls, petty theft and generally passive behaviours (Berne, 1961).

TA and the climate within an organization

There is much talk of climates within organizations and how the climate affects staff working within them. The study of TA can make us appreciate just how as managers we create a critical parent or more adult climate in our many and varied transactions with our colleagues, staff, patients and clients. For instance, how do you and other managers in your workplace deal with the issue of telephone calls made by your staff ? Do you forbid them, get them to tell the switchboard that it is not personal, allow local personal calls, tell them at intervals what the phone bill is and how much is being spent? You can see the potential here for parent–child and adult–adult transactions.

Stroking

The other aspect we would like to draw your attention to in this short survey of TA is the notion of stroking. A stroke is a sign of recognition; it is the giving and receiving of positive strokes that develop emotionally healthy people with a feeling of confidence in themselves, a general feeling of being 'OK'. Strokes are powerful. One way of making use of TA is to examine your pattern of giving strokes. Do you say 'thank you' enough to staff? Do you make constructive comments on their work, praising those parts which deserve praise and making helpful comments on those aspects which need to be improved? Have you ever received back from a manager a report that took you ages to complete which is either covered with red ink or has no marks on it at all? These are examples of negative strokes and they can cause hurt.'Well if that's all they feel about my work I won't be so forthcoming next time.'

We could all do with reviewing our stroking behaviours. Our manager in the first appraisal situation gave out a number of very negative strokes: his tone, his lack of non-verbal greeting, his accusatory language and his dismissal of the positive aspects of the staff member's performance as shown in her supervisor's reports. Do you ever perform like that? Do you give out enough strokes – positive ones? If we were to ask your staff the last time you had thanked them personally for something they had done would we be able to find plenty of examples?

There was an account in the *Scotsman* newspaper of executives being sent on courses to teach them how to say 'thank you' in the most appropriate way to their staff. Maybe this is something we should all take more seriously?

Becoming a more effective communicator

Much of the material in this chapter you were probably already aware of, some may have been new. The key question is: how can I become more effective in terms of my interpersonal communication skills? Well, we certainly hope our advice will be useful, we have included a number of key texts on communication which we recommend. One of the most practical things you could do is to take a more active interest in communication that you see practised round you. Who are the people who are respected for their management of meetings? Who issues readable memos and reports; who has the reputation for being a fair and open interviewer? Very often there is a pool of hidden talent in organizations; such people could be used for coaching of staff, even running short courses. And talking of courses there are very many providers in the market who will be happy to run one for you and your colleagues or staff. A word of caution: do make sure that any such provider understands your particular needs and they do not just pull a course in general communication skills off the shelf.

Conclusion

This chapter has outlined a number of aspects of interpersonal skills that managers need to be aware of in their work. We have not had the space to include written communication and do more than sketch in non-verbal communication. We refer you to texts which we think do cover these areas well and to others that amplify the material – notably on TA – which we have discussed in this chapter. A great deal of evidence on the criteria for successful organizations, be they public or private, has come down to the crucial importance of managers being effective communicators. So often managers are promoted and not given much help with these skills – they are assumed to have them. We hope that your reading of this material and thinking round the ideas outlined will inform you and your colleagues of good practice.

References

Anderson A, Brown G and Yule G (1985) *Listening Skills*. Scottish Education Dept., Edinburgh.
Audit Commission (1993) *Trusting in the Future*. HMSO, London.
Berne E (1961) *Transactional Analysis*. Evergreen Press, London.
Goodworth C T (1985) *Effective Interviewing*. Business Books, London.
Statt D (1994) *The Psychology of Work*. Macmillan, London.

Further reading

Dimbleby R and Burton G (1990) *Beyond Words*. Edward Arnold, London.
Ellis R and McClintock A (1994) *If You Take My Meaning*. Edward Arnold, London.
Harris T A (1970) *I'm OK – You're OK*. Pan Books, London.

5

The manager as leader

In this chapter we examine various approaches to leadership: we provide definitions of manager, administrator and leader; we survey the qualities, styles, skills, situational and action-centred approaches to leadership. We suggest that successful leaders are those that pay close attention to the relationships they have with those they lead.

Introduction

This area has received a great deal of attention recently. Numerous books have been written and analyses produced on the question of leadership. The quality of leadership is of very great concern to the future of health and social care services. Finding the right people to lead an organization is of enormous importance to the success of that organization. As we shall see often in this book, the increasing importance given to devolved management requires a more flexible kind of leadership.

One of the problems is that there is often confusion between the terms leadership and management. They are often used synonymously. Then there is administration; where does that fit into the picture? Is that different from managing or is it a part of the management process? And can administrators be leaders? Even if we agree on definitions, the questions arise: How do we find leaders? How do we recruit them and train them? Let us begin with some definitions.

Administrator

An administrator, as defined by the Collins Cobuild Dictionary, is a person whose job involves helping to organize and supervise the way that a company, institution or other organization is run.

This, we suggest, is about the necessary chores involved in making things work, seeing to it that procedures are carried out, that no blockages occur in the smooth working of the ward, the department, the unit. This is an important part of any manager's job; however, the danger is that it can become the job itself.

We saw in Chapter 2, in our overview of management, the importance of delegation. If the manager is unable, or unwilling to delegate then he or she will find the job becoming all administration and there will not be enough time for management. Administration is that part of the management task that can be most easily delegated.

Manager

According to the dictionary, the term 'to manage' can be defined by the statement: 'If you manage an organization, business, system etc., you are responsible for controlling it'.

This implies that the manager is able to steer the ship, to keep all the crew moving in the right direction, to oversee the whole picture. Managing implies being able to keep abreast of what is happening.

Let us now look at the ingredients of a successful manager.

Activity

What do you think are the chief ingredients of a successful manager. Jot down a few ideas before you continue reading.

The Management Charter Initiative (1990) says that to be a successful manager you need to be good at:

- showing a concern for excellence;
- setting and prioritizing objectives;
- monitoring/responding to actual as against planned activities;
- showing sensitivity to the needs of others;
- obtaining the commitment of others;
- presenting oneself positively to others;
- showing self confidence and personal drive;
- managing personal emotions and stress;
- managing personal learning and development;
- collecting and organizing information;
- identifying and applying concepts; and
- taking decisions.

For comparison, in *A Manager's Guide to Self Development*, Pedler *et al.* (1994) state that a successful manager needs to show:

- command of basic facts/relevant professional understanding;
- continuing sensitivity to events;

- analytical, problem-solving, decision-making skills;
- social skills and abilities;
- emotional resilience;
- pro-activity: inclination to respond purposely to events;
- creativity;
- mental agility;
- balanced learning habits and skills; and
- self knowledge.

How was your list? Did it include many of these ingredients? Much of the way we see management will depend on own experiences; the kinds of manager we have worked for.

Well, are we any further forward in finding out what *leadership* is? Is it the sum of all these attributes or it something extra – something different, a special set of qualities? Our dictionary is not so helpful, it merely states: 'Leadership, the qualities that make someone a good leader; for example, the ability to make decisions, give orders and gain other people's respect and trust.'

There is widespread belief that leaders are those who *transform*, i.e. change the direction of the organization and take the staff along with them, while managers are those who merely *transact* the business, keeping things steady as they are – static rather than dynamic orientation.

Leadership according to this view appears to be that quality, returning to the previous metaphor, of not only steering the ship, but also taking it into deeper waters, if necessary changing course and taking the crew with you. According to this view, leadership implies some attempt to move things, to change things, to provide vision and direction to an organization.

Many organizations have their mission statements: leaders, one could argue, are those individuals who make such statements happen, who make the vision real. Crucially here is the ability of this person to communicate to those 'led' what the 'transformation' is all about. The danger with a trans-forming leader is that many are left behind in the dark. We shall see an example of this in our first case study later in this chapter (page 67).

Styles

There has been considerable research into whether 'democratic', 'autocratic' or '*laissez-faire*' styles of leadership produce the best results. Most research suggests that the democratic style gets the best results. This means letting people in on the task, listening to people's ideas, allowing groups to work with a certain measure of freedom in the way the task is done, it is the 'adult–adult' TA approach we saw in the last chapter. However, there appear to be some situations where a more autocratic style can achieve better results. This is where the task is simple, repetitive, where those involved know what they want and simply need to be told, 'OK please get on with it'.

There are real difficulties facing leaders who champion the democratic style: either those being led do not recognize it as being democratic or, because most organizations are hierarchical in structure, democracy may dwindle and old patterns of command renew themselves. There have been very many examples where this has happened, you may have witnessed this yourself. It may be that the only approach is to follow the example of Ricardo Semler in Brazil and completely transform the structure. His staff decide on who gets which job, who gets what pay and holidays; the total marketing, advertising and approach to investment and training is democratically organized. Unless we are prepared to restructure our organizations then the best we can hope for may well be to make sure that our leadership is based on sound communication with those we lead, that their ideas are listened to and that we all work hard on building up good working relationships. We shall see more about this in the next chapter on groups and team building.

Qualities

A number of studies of leadership have focused on specific qualities, such as those in the lists above. Qualities inevitably lead us to consider personality. A survey of research by Statt (1994) found that three qualities appear to be significant:

- Intelligence
- Tolerance for ambiguity
- Self image.

Effective leaders appear to need a little more intelligence that those whom they lead (however too great a gap in intelligence between led and leader can produce problems). The research also suggests that such leaders can hold opposing views, consider various options and that they are confident about themselves, possessing a positive image of themselves and their abilities. We should not be surprised at these particular qualities. It is very difficult to lead unless one has a positive (but not arrogant) feeling about oneself, is at least as bright as those one is leading and is able to consider various views and not be blinkered towards one course of action.

We may want to consider these when judging potential for leadership, but it can never be the total answer for a number of reasons:

- It is very difficult to get people to agree as to what precisely are those qualities that we wish for a manager in the health or social services.
- The need for certain qualities changes over time. It may be that particular qualities of drive and determination which were considered essential in the 1960s are not so desirable in the complex world of the 1990s where we have to build co-operation and consensus rather than impose it.
- More people are needed as leaders than ever before. The increasing trend to devolved management structures in health and social care will mean

that many more leaders have to be found, and the scale of their leadership may be reduced to a ward or a team rather than a whole hospital or centre, but the skills are the same.

This is not to say that the qualities approach has been rejected. Many of you reading this would subscribe to a number of those ingredients on the two lists presented. We know that managers have to have some degree of intelligence and alertness and the ability to restrain their own feelings and emotions from interfering with decision making.

Skills

From the two lists on pages 61 and 62 we can identify a number of specific skills that are needed by any manager. In this we could include the ability:

- to present a case with confidence and within clear structures;
- to read and interpret balance sheets and costs structures;
- to write clearly and to summarize key points from documents, interviews and meetings;
- to be able to chair meetings;
- to be able to listen in an open, non-judgmental way;
- to be able to negotiate; and
- to be able to manage time.

As with the issue of qualities it is very difficult to get people to agree on what should be in such a list.

Activity

In thinking of managers you have worked for – and are now working under – what other skills would you place on our list?

Situational models

Leadership, according to this view, is all about how people in authority learn to handle situations and from this experience go on to become better at leading others.

A great deal of the learning behind many MBA programmes lies in the keeping of 'reflective logs', reflecting about theory when dealing with practice. Kolb (1971) suggests an Experiential Learning Model as shown in Figure 5.1. According to this model leaders can develop their leadership skills and abilities by becoming reflective. Pedlar et al. (1994) put this in a very simple way as shown in Figure 5.2.

As we wrote in our introduction, this book is based very much on the premise that reflective learning is necessary and useful – hence the inclusion

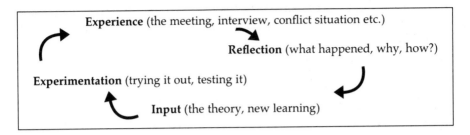

Figure 5.1 Diagrammatic representation of Kolb's experiential learning model.

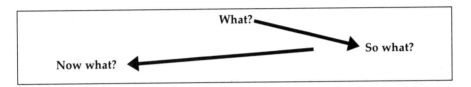

Figure 5.2 Reflective learning.

of case studies and activities. A manager who does not reflect upon past failures and successes may never become an effective leader.

Action-centred leadership

A third model of leadership is provided by action-centred leadership (ACL), based upon work by John Adair (1979) who has written extensively on leadership theory and practice. This approach involves three interrelated but highly distinctive requirements of a leader. These are:

- to define and achieve the task;
- to build up and co-ordinate a team to do this; and
- to satisfy the individuals within the team.

He suggests that we can break these three into their various needs:

- *Task needs.* The difference between a team and a collection of individuals is that the team usually has common purposes, aims, goals.
- *Team needs.* In order to achieve these objectives, the group needs to be held together. This will require that conflicts are resolved, individual roles clarified within the team and a measure of consensus arrived at as to how the team achieves its ends.
- *Individual needs.* Within any group, individuals will also have their own needs. They will need to know what their roles are, lines of responsibility,

an opportunity to be challenged, to be rewarded with praise and appraised fairly on performance.

The leader in ACL

The leader's task is to try to satisfy all three areas of need by achieving the task, building the team and satisfying individual needs. There are problems if the leader concentrates on the task to the exclusion of all else, for instance going all out to improve financial control while neglecting the training, encouragement and communication with the members of the group he or she is managing. Likewise it would not be profitable to spend too much time creating team spirit while neglecting the task and the needs of the individuals in the team. So, according to Adair, the leader must try to achieve balance by acting in all three areas of overlapping needs. This can be illustrated as shown in Figure 5.3.

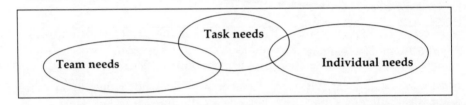

Figure 5.3 The three overlapping needs in the action-centred leadership model.

Table 5.1 summarizes the range of responsibilities taken on by any leader. Some of these are fairly obvious. For example, planning is a key attribute for all managers which we identified under planning, implementation and evaluation (PIE). But notice the stress here given to the support and control function; it is one thing to set up the team and identify individual and team needs, it is another quite separate and equally important task to be able to 'recognize, encourage and enthuse' to keep the team feeling that you care and are involved.

Perhaps this is one of the key differences between management and leadership and shows how one shades into the other: leadership builds a team so that there is care, the individuals feel that this leader actually cares for their success and is not simply managing them as individual units. Communication, one of the central functions on the Adair checklist, is all about getting the appropriate message to the appropriate individuals so that they can perform their job better in the team. Leaders communicate not only to inform but to show that they 'care' in the widest sense of the word: care when things go right as well as when they go wrong, care enough to show interest in performance, care enough to demonstrate involvement and engagement, care enough to spare time from busy schedules to find out what is happening and communicate this with others who should know.

Table 5.1 Leadership checklist

Function	Task	Team	Individual needs
Define objectives	Identify task and constraints	Set targets, involve team	Set targets and responsibilities
Plan	Establish resources and decide priorities	Structure and delegate	Assess skills, train
Communicate	Brief and check understanding	Consult and obtain feedback	Listen, advise, enthuse
Support and control	Monitor progress, check standards	Co-ordinate, reconcile conflict	Recognize, encourage, counsel
Evaluate	Review, replan, summarize	Reward success, learn from failure	Appraise and guide

Effective leadership is so much a matter of building effective relationships. We examined the manager as communicator in Chapter 4; now let us see what can happen when relationships are not built sufficiently.

Case study 5.1

Robert is an experienced hill walker who has been asked to take a party on the Southern Upland Way walk across the Borders Region of Scotland. The party is formed from members of local ramblers' clubs. They all meet in a local pub and Robert runs over the aim of the expedition. *(Defines objectives)*

He tells them the kind of schedule he intends to keep and also informs them of the constraints in terms of harshness of terrain, expected weather conditions, provision of bed and breakfast accommodation, etc. Despite the keenness of the party there is some disquiet as to the proposed route and the heavy demands that will be made on them. Some of the older ones say that they will probably leave the main party after a couple of days – they do not think they will want to do more than that. *(Plan – establishing resources, assessing skills)*

The walk starts, the weather is worse than expected and the route far more severe than the impression given in the pub. The older ones start to fall behind. Robert believes that a good pace has to be maintained and leads from the front. *(Communicate – listen, consult)*

Into the second day some of the party are getting a little depressed by the pace being set, the poor weather and the steepness of much of the ground. Robert is surprised at the amount of dissent in the party. He made it clear the previous day that if the pace fell too far behind the schedule then a number of bed and breakfast bookings would be lost; he had been asked to lead a party to walk the Southern Upland Way, not go for the normal Sunday afternoon ramble. *(Support/control – encourage, counsel, reconcile conflict)*

The next day a number of the party decide not to proceed with the walk; there is some feeling that they have been let down by Robert, their leader. The remainder elect to go on. The walk proceeds and finally reaches its destination. The party thank Robert for his time and effort. He decides not to undertake another such journey with such a large party, it was all too much effort. *(Evaluate – review, replan, appraise, learn from failure)*

You may have been on such a walk with such a leader. Can we really use the term 'leader' with him? He did not demonstrate many of the facets of leadership we have been examining. Following the Adair model he failed on many accounts. He did not show sufficient *care* for his team; he failed to weld the individuals into a team – all with a common purpose, *a clear goal*. He failed to *consult and listen*, so that yes he was leading from the front but what was he leading? Good leaders operate not only from the front but they also come alongside and support the stragglers. This is showing care.

A leader is someone people will follow; some kind of understanding has been achieved – almost a contract between leaders and led has been made. This stimulating hike developed into an endurance race, no real contract or understanding had been achieved. Furthermore, at the end there was no attempt to reflect on failure and see how to learn from it. Now compare Case study 5.2.

Case study 5.2

A senior nurse has been appointed to head up a group which is investigating the training needs of her staff group (a training needs analysis) (Task). She forms a small team representing all sections and levels from the staff (Team). She briefs the individual members of the team as to their respective roles within the group (Individuals). At a meeting with the whole group she clarifies the nature of the remit including the time constraints and desired targets. *(Define objectives)*

With the group she sets about establishing resources (time, access to support staff, etc.). She decides on the structure of the TNA and with the members of the group sets out delegation of responsibilities, including hers. At the same time she is conscious that not all members of her team will be able to undertake the work of questionnaire design, inter-viewing, job shadowing and observation without some training and skill enhancement. She is able to negotiate some training sessions for such members. *(Plan)*

Because of the size of this project she sends out a weekly bulletin to all the members of the project to keep them informed as to progress. She also meets with team leaders and whenever she can talks with individuals working on the project. *(Communicate)*

At the end of the first week of the TNA she calls team leaders together for a review meeting. She hears about certain difficulties with senior staff not agreeing to give time. She agrees to meet these staff and after some negotiation smoothes the problem out. The project team feel much happier when she is able to inform them of this. *(Support and control)*

When the project is completed and the data collected, she gets as many of the team as possible to join with her in a review. This is very open. Basically she asks the group to list for her all those features of the project and the way it was organized and managed which were positive, which they enjoyed, and all those which could have been improved. They do this on a flip chart. The discussion is very frank and many ideas, especially about the way in which the team were trained in interviewing skills and the way in which the data were collected for the final report, were criticized. *(Evaluation)*

We can see from these case studies why Adair called his approach to leadership 'Action Centred'. The leader in Case study 5.1 was not in the centre; he led from the front it is true but he was never at the centre of planning, checking, enthusing, caring, evaluating – and all the other functions on our checklist. When the going got tough the tough stopped going – to misquote a well-known phrase. There was no 'contract' and not enough real care.

In Case study 5.2 our senior nurse provided a structured approach to her leadership of that project. At some times she directly involved herself – as when she had to negotiate for training – at other times she kept further to the sidelines, but still progressed through the various stages from definition of task to evaluation of performance. We saw in Chapter 2 that managers have to be flexible in responding to situations. The Adair model fully incorporates such flexibility, but this is not at the expense of following through a structure that the Adair checklist provides.

We will see from Chapter 6 that if any team is to function effectively then *all* the 'players' must understand the objectives and their role in the 'game plan'. This takes us back to our last chapter where we emphasized the importance of role clarification both individually and within the team. If you can only see your own bit of the project then it is unlikely that you will feel very committed to any outcome: your horizon will be limited. This is perhaps the greatest challenge of team building: to get even those with the humblest role to feel fully involved, to open up for them a horizon.

We have briefly surveyed various approaches to leadership: the *qualities,* where we identified a number of significant characteristics, the *skills* which a leader will need, and the *situational,* where we have said that effective leaders behave according to the situation. Finally, we looked at the *action-centred approach,* where the leader places himself or herself at the centre of operations to build individuals into a team to perform the task.

References

Adair J (1979) *Action Centred Leadership.* Gower, Aldershot.
Kolb D (1971) *Organisational Psychology.* Prentice Hall, London.
Management Charter Initiative (1990) *Management Standards Implementation Pack.* London.
Pedler M, Burgoyne J and Boydell T (1994) *A Manager's Guide to Self Development.* McGraw-Hill, London.
Statt D (1994) *The Psychology of Work.* Macmillan, London.

Further reading

Adair J (1984) *The Skills of Leadership.* Gower, Aldershot.
Harvey Jones J (1989) *Making it Happen.* Fontana, London.
Semler R (1994) *Maverick.* Arrow Press, London.

6

The manager as group leader and team builder

In this chapter we deal with the manager as group leader and team builder. This aspect of management is receiving increased attention. We look at various models of how groups behave and some of the dangers to their development. Key aspects of chairing are also outlined.

'You're only as good as your team.'
'If you want to find out how good a leader she is, ask her team.'
'Who would take over your section? I mean supposing you were ill?'
'All gone out to lunch. Team building eh? Someone's birthday eh?'
'He's very brilliant but he's got to realize that we haven't got time for prima donnas here. You've got to get him to work with the rest of us.'
'We're devolving more financial responsibilities to your team.'

Introduction

What constitutes a good team leader?

All these comments refer to teams and their leaders. We saw in the last chapter that ideas of what constitutes a good leader have changed somewhat over recent years. We are no longer looking for isolated, aloof and brilliant individuals striding out well in front of their subordinates, flag in hand looking back to see who, if anyone, is following behind. What is needed now is a leader who can work with people, build a team, harness individual talents into a collective effort. We need leaders who can motivate and inspire and who have the necessary vision to lead from the front. Leadership is extremely difficult: it is an art. Few of us have all the necessary qualities. The crucial question is can such a manager carry the team with him or her? Vision by itself is an important asset but the crucial component is that ability to 'sell' it to the members of the team and move them towards successful completion of the task.

In a sports team the captain is there to encourage the development of a strategy by tapping ideas from the players – the game plan – to communicate this clearly to the players, to stimulate, inspire and generally be there to encourage and support individuals. Team can mean Together Each Achieves More, or it can mean Terrible Effort: All Mayhem, or even Terrible Effort: All Moaning!

We have already examined the action-centred model, in which the leader is at the centre, taking care of the individual and bringing him or her into the team; now let us examine another challenge.

Keeping talented individuals in the team

One of the greatest challenges for managers is to prevent talented individuals from leaving, flying off to greener pastures, setting themselves up in direct competition, or becoming increasingly demotivated, their talents rusting and their productivity falling. We mentioned the concept of 'rust out' in Chapter 3. You may have experienced it: the situation where one is not being challenged, there is no sense of stretching the job and you feel you are literally rusting away, your talents not being used.

It is equally important that people are not smothered by the inertia, the very security and orthodoxy of the group. Peters (1992) has suggested that one of the features of a leader is not to organize but to disorganize, in other words to go out and prevent people from getting too cosy and demotivated, to reform systems and break inertia as soon as it becomes obvious that a group has become too set and comfortable in its ways. The only solution may be to break it up and start again with a clean sheet of paper. Such a move will cause conflict and create angst but that is better than a slow atrophying of talent and ability and a waste of resources. We have seen in Chapter 2 how change must be managed; if it is not then there are painful consequences for those involved. As manager you have wider responsibilities – to other staff, to customers, patients and colleagues. One group's comfort and security cannot be allowed to stand in the way of the needs of the organization.

Some general approaches to groups

Here we outline some of the theoretical approaches in our understanding of groups and their behaviour. Space only permits us to mention some of the more well-known and obvious theories here. You will find others in the suggested further reading at the end of the chapter.

Tuckman's model

Managers often find themselves puzzled and disappointed by the inability of the group they are managing to work to deadlines, produce work of sufficient quality and sustain any kind of motivation. Tuckman (1965) suggested that one of the principal reasons that groups fail is that they do not progress through the necessary stages. He identified five distinct stages: forming, storming, norming, performing and adjournment, and put forward the idea that groups can get stuck at any point on this progression, failing to make headway.

Forming

The group starts off, boundaries are explored, there is interest in how each member of the group stands in relation to the leader, there is the process of settling down to the task.

Storming

This is the stage where troubles may occur, tensions arise over procedures, the remit of the group, time allocations, deadlines and the nature of individual roles within the team. Tuckman suggests that this is a very necessary and even healthy phase and those groups that do not enter into a vigorous 'storming' do not go on to thrive. It is at this stage that the leader has to take on the Adair (1986) model and build the individuals into a team. It is much better that conflict arises at this stage and is allowed to come into the open where it can be dealt with, rather than festering, only to erupt at a critical moment in the project.

Conflict is so often regarded as a negative – a purely destructive process. However we could consider some conflict, the storming processes, as being constructive conflict. It is often only by storming through these conflicts that the group emerges at the other end more healthy, more sure of respective roles – yours as manager included – and its overall remit.

You may have had experience of being in a group which appeared to be working at only half power and this may have been because of a lack of clarity over these matters.

We can see this happening during meetings. We look around and notice the puzzled faces – people not sure as to why they are sitting there. It is essential that the leader confronts this situation and clarifies the positions and individuals' roles in the group. However at the same time we need to take care not to stifle the initiative, to make the role description too tight and restrictive. There is always the tension between wanting to provide a clear remit and straight-jacketing the individual or the group so that initiative and creativity are lost and opportunities missed.

Norming

The members of the group have a clear sense of where they want to go; the leader has helped them to clarify their positions. They agree, usually after much discussion, on the essential *ground rules*.

Performing

Here the group will be self motivated and interested in concentrating on the job at hand. The leader's role is to, where necessary, guide, motivate the individual members and assist in the co-ordination of the work of the group. Sometimes the leader's role when all the team is busy will be to go and buy them all fish and chips, or at least to get out of their way.

Adjournment or disbandment

This is the final stage. The task has been done, the job achieved and the leader's role now is to carry the members of the team into a new task: to allow for a time of loss and to motivate them for new endeavours. Before this happens it is important for the leader to thank individuals and celebrate the completion of the task.

Activity

Read Case study 6.1. Decide what actions the leader (Susan) could have taken, bearing in mind Tuckman's advice.

Case study 6.1

Susan's boss has asked her to put together a project group which she wants to use to monitor absenteeism within the health care organization in which they work. There is concern that staff absenteeism has been increasing and that not enough has been done to combat it. As a first stage it is essential to monitor what is actually happening and to come up with a policy that will have general support within the organization. This project group has representatives from all the various departments and sections of the organization. Susan has been asked to be its convenor and get the ball rolling. Senior management would like to have some definite ideas and recommendations before the end of the year. It is now late October.

Susan writes to all those on the list provided for her by her manager. She invites them to a first meeting in her office for the afternoon of Thursday 26 October. She realizes when she is drafting this notice that she does not know some of the participants very well and she feels less than 100 per cent sure as to the remit. She tries rather late in the day to get an interview with her boss but finds she is away for the week on a course. At the meeting which gathers on the Thursday, Susan outlines the remit of the group as given to her by her boss and asks for ideas. Susan begins to write up on a flip chart the various ideas. They agree to examine these and return a week later for a more focused discussion.

A week later and Susan notices that two members are not there – despite everyone having cleared their diaries the week before. As the meeting gets going, and various ideas are discussed, Susan notices that there is a lack of enthusiasm and a fair bit of muttering around the table. She tries to concentrate the group's thoughts and suggests that a subcommittee is formed to take the issues forward and report back to the full group within a month. This suggestion is given lukewarm support. Susan when meeting with her manager later in the week confesses that she feels the group has not gelled, that their enthusiasm for the project has dulled and that some of them seem to be not very co-operative. The manager listens with some impatience and decides that she ought to attend the next meeting of the full group to move things on.

At this meeting there is a fair amount of tension and aggression. A number of the committee complain to the manager that they were not fully informed at the start of the proceedings and that had they known the nature of the task they would have had a great deal more to say.

Responsibilities for this failure could be laid at Susan's and her manager's door. Her manager should have briefed her more thoroughly; however remember the point we made in Chapter 4 as to where responsibilities for communication lie. We suggested that the listener has a very real responsibility to check and amplify the communication being received. Susan should have encouraged a 'storming' stage with the group, encouraging open discussion of their remit. Some healthy conflict at this first meeting would have helped to clear the air and prevent people brooding and then blocking progress, as happened at their second meeting. This is a very good example of what Tuckman would call a 'failure to storm'. Susan naturally was anxious to get the project group off to a positive start. She knew that her manager was keen to see progress. She had been handed the brief and so pressed on, but at some cost. The formation of subcommittees at this time is putting the cart before the horse. It is as though it is only when a group has broken through the turbulence that it can move into quieter, smoother waters.

Group think and conformity

The second general approach to groups consists of theories relating to group think and conformity. You may have come across this latter phenomenon. It arises where one member of a group – very often the leader or chair – because of his or her personality, position, ability to reward or punish, creates an atmosphere which discourages participants from fully expressing their views, particularly criticisms of the leader.

How can managers who lead/chair reduce the chances of conformity happening?

One very simple but effective rule is for the leader of any group not to present his or her ideas or suggestions at the start of discussion but to allow others to have their say. The key role here is that of the facilitator: listening to individuals, eliciting responses from them and summing up at intervals. The difficulty is that once the leader has spoken it can become increasingly difficult for others to be critical and to express their true feelings in his or her presence. Hence there can be a great deal of conformity – apparent rather than real – at many meetings. We may ask why have meetings unless there is some measure of frank and open discussion, unless we want to follow a more Japanese way of doing things in which very often the meeting is concerned with ceremony and the disagreements and exchange of views has happened beforehand?

One practical way in which we can prevent conformity from arising in groups and therefore a lack of frank and open speaking is to encourage regular discussions on process, i.e. how we are doing as opposed to what we are doing. Very often these discussions can go better if we take the members of the group away from their normal day-to-day surroundings and concerns, an away day or afternoon, without telephones ringing and colleagues knocking at the door.

We have found that it is useful for the manager on these occasions to set the discussion going with the group along the lines:

What do we *like* about the way we work together as a group?
What do we think could be *improved*?

Sometimes it might be better for the leader to absent him or herself from the discussions so as to allow more frank speaking, but there are merits in this being a whole group affair where positive criticism is provided.

In a way it links with the idea of upward appraisal, which we discuss in Chapter 14.

Another aspect of managing groups we should consider has been described as 'groupthink'. Janis (1972) defines this using the following description.

> When a group of people who respect each other's opinions arrives at a unanimous view, each member is likely to feel that the belief must be true. This reliance on consensus validation tends to replace individual critical thinking and reality testing unless there are clear cut disagreements among the members. The members of a face-to-face group often become inclined, without realising it, to prevent latent disagreement from surfacing, when they are about to initiate a risky course of action.

Can you think of a time when you felt groupthink was a problem with the group of which you were a member/leader?

You will probably have experienced some of the symptoms described by Janis: 'a view that each member is likely to feel that the belief (decision) must be true'. The question is what do we do about it? How do we ginger up the group before the disease gets a grip?

Our suggested approach is one in which the leader seeks to bring in some fresh air to the group; this, we believe, can help improve the general morale and climate, so increasing a feeling of trust and the chance that everyone in the group will feel more free to speak his or her mind. This is in line with the tenets of Transactional Analysis. We suggested in Chapter 4 that in our working relationships we should be moving to adult–adult transactions.

Providing an effective mixture in your team

This is extremely important when it comes to giving and receiving criticism without it being hurtful or vindictive, thus causing resentment and ill feeling. This approach, in which we concentrate first on the positive and then on those aspects that could be improved is very much geared to establishing and maintaining an adult–adult approach.

Belbin (1981) suggests that what groups need is a mixture of 'types'. He argues that we bring two distinct roles to a team: our *technical role* (our particular expertise) and our *team role* (what we contribute to the success of the team's effort). Belbin has spent many years investigating why teams fail, and having exhausted the usual parameters suggests that very often there have not been sufficient team roles represented. Table 6.1 shows a selection of the team types he identified.

Table 6.1 Some of the team types identified by Belbin

Team type	Typical features	Plus qualities	Allowable weakness
Shaper	Highly strung	Drive, energy	Impatience
Plant	Unorthodox	Imagination	Up in the clouds
Completer finisher	Painstaking	Perfectionist	Worrier
Chairman	Calm/controlled	Sense of objectives	Not over-creative

Belbin has for a long time argued that we need to encourage a wide representation of type to be included in any group that we are setting up from scratch. This is one of the ways we can avoid the perils of groupthink.

Notice how he sets out the plus qualities of each type. How many of us have regretted that there was no 'completer finisher' in the group to tie up the loose ends, or a 'plant' who could spark off good ideas, come up with unusual angles to a problem, ask the simple but penetrating question and cause us all to think long and hard? (The reason why Belbin called this type a 'plant' is that he discovered that very often a group was underfunctioning because it did not have such a person who would provide creative thinking.)

Allowable weaknesses

Notice that Belbin, apart from displaying the positive features, also gives us the downside, the allowable weaknesses. You may have had someone in your group who although excellent at thinking up new approaches and bursting into life with stimulating episodes of lateral thinking, was also on occasions, 'a bit of a pain in the neck', doodling on the committee minutes and gazing out of the window instead of concentrating on the matters in hand. This is the price we may have to pay for the 'plant'. Belbin suggests that as group members and leaders we all contribute various strengths and deficits as team members and that is apart from any technical expertise we bring.

Applications of the Belbin approach

Of course this is all very well if you are building a team up from scratch; you can look around and, subject to normal constraints, try and select a number of these types. (Belbin has produced a number of assessments of type; you may wish to try them out on yourself and colleagues to see what preferred team type is indicated for you.) But what happens if you take over the running of an existing team?

First, we would say that the climate, the atmosphere in which the team operates is crucial for bringing out what already exists in the way of team type; this may be inhibited by overdominant leading, lack of confidence amongst participants as to their roles and the terms of reference of the group – all the factors we have already noted.

The leader's role as facilitator is crucial in ensuring that members are encouraged to speak and contribute their ideas in an atmosphere which is conducive to genuine openness and frank speaking. 'Plants' will not reveal their creative thinking process if they fear they will be squashed and their ideas ridiculed by others. The leader has to make sure that the ground rules are quite clear as to this point. Good manners, consideration for others and attentive listening need to be encouraged. This is what brainstorming can be so useful for, it releases the plants' abilities. The rules of brainstorming should protect individuals from having their ideas ridiculed.

Generally we should avoid taking on those roles (such as completer finisher) for which we have neither appetite nor competence. However, it is very likely that we have more than one preferred role, and there may well be a need for us to play more than one role particularly within a small group.

Chairing

One of the interesting aspects of Belbin's work is the notion that perhaps not all leaders should be chairing their groups. As one might expect, many leaders display pronounced 'shaper' qualities: drive, readiness to challenge inertia, qualities which might make them less comfortable in a facilitation, chairing role. Belbin has a 'chairman' as one team type (*see* Table 6.1). You can see that this type has much to offer to the group. Whereas the 'shaper' may certainly get the meeting completed on time, he or she may also steamroller proceedings and, determined to push ahead, not allow contributions from the other team types to emerge as they should.

There are many books on the market which cover the chairing of meetings very well. We refer you to some of these at the end of the chapter. What follows is a rapid survey of some of the key skills and approaches to chairing we think will be of assistance to you in your work with colleagues, staff and patients.

Planning

Start the meeting by *planning* well beforehand. Plan for the time you have at your disposal and the time you think you will need. There is a tendency for meetings to follow Parkinson's principle: meetings expand to fill the time available for their completion! Normally, the more time that we can spend planning for the meeting, the better it will go.

When members of a group see the list of items on the agenda there should be few surprises. Try to get the group to take 'ownership' of the agenda. Negotiate with the group at the start of the meeting what kind of time allocation per subject would be reasonable, bearing in mind a finishing time which all can agree on. One of the most obvious and successful ways of controlling a meeting is to get the group to agree on the available time for the meeting and then keep reminding them as the meeting proceeds how much is left. Use comments such as, 'We've already taken ten minutes over this issue, I certainly don't want to cut what could be a promising discussion but I should point out that at this rate we will not be able to complete all the agenda we set out for ourselves.'

Alertness

One of the key aspects of chairing any meeting is *keeping alert*. Keeping an eye on the clock and noticing how time is passing is one aspect of alertness, another is keeping watch on the non-verbal communication, the leakage of those sitting round the table (or standing up if you are following advice from Japanese organizations to keep the meeting short). Knowing your members of the group can assist in this process of alertness since the chair has to keep in mind the 'technical roles' of members, knowing who has 'expertise' in what particular areas and who to invite into which part of the discussion. Chairpersons need to take care when calling for contributions: it can sound like a touch of discipline: 'Harry', can mean, 'hey wake up there please'. It is probably better to look around the table and say: 'How does the group feel about this...Harry?' This enables everyone to enter into the discussion and also allows the chairperson to bring in people he or she knows have something to say.

Alertness also means watching out for the inevitable moments when the meeting begins to *drift off* the point in question. It can happen so easily and before you know where you are people are talking about something which, although interesting, is off the agenda and should be kept either for the coffee break or later in the meeting.

You have to make sure that everyone is speaking to the point. Catch wanderers before they go too far. It is much easier to bring people back to the point if this is done quickly; once you allow someone to ramble on and off the point, bringing him or her back can be very difficult indeed. They have tasted freedom and often refuse to be roped in! The whole balance of the meeting will tilt towards the interests of the one person speaking and others may well get irritated and stop listening or start trying to break in. All this will undermine your authority and weaken the established procedures of the meeting. Remember that one of the key functions of a meeting is to allow equal access to participation. If one person hogs it all then others will have less opportunity to break through. They will then be more likely to break the rules and 'mutiny'.

Being alert also means checking to see that everyone around the table *has understood* what is being said. Often participants will not ask questions because they do not want to appear to be stupid. It is your job as chairperson to see that people do understand.

Activity

How can you achieve this at your meetings? Reflect on this before you continue reading.

A list of strategies designed to ensure that everyone in a meeting has understood could include the following.

- Ask for a summary if someone has made a lengthy contribution.
- Get them to summarize the key points. If someone is to make a presentation to the group, it is a good idea for them to list the key points on a single sheet of paper.
- Provide a summary. After a number of contributions it is useful for the chairperson to summarize the key points. These summaries are also useful to the person taking the notes/minutes. You can assist this process by writing key points on a flip chart. If you delegate this task do make sure that the person doing the writing up (a) actually paraphrases the

contributions correctly and (b) is able to stop writing to take part in the discussion.

- Paraphrase and check back for understanding. Sometimes what participants say is not very clearly expressed or focused for all kinds of reasons – nerves, getting genuinely muddled, handling a difficult concept that needs more thinking time, etc. The chairperson needs to keep alert for this and try to clarify: 'I'm not sure I've got that Susan. Are you saying that we should...?'
- Look around the group at the non-verbal communication. This should give you a good clue as to whether or not contributions are being understood and if some paraphrasing and checking back is required.

Rules

We have already looked at some aspects of control through the negotiation and management of the time allocated for the meeting. Being alert as chairperson is an essential part of being in control. The essence of a meeting is that discussion takes place under rules. These need to be established during the 'storming' stage and must not be left to vague assumptions. Members need to feel that they are protected by the rules.

Activity

What kind of rules would you think ought to be established for meetings whether formal or informal ? Reflect on this before continuing.

Some common rules for meetings are that:

- members can say things in confidence within the group;
- members will not be 'squashed' by older, louder, more senior members just when they are about to say something;
- members' ideas will be recorded and not left hanging; and
- members' ideas will not be ridiculed or dismissed without due care and consideration.

We often consider that these kinds of chairing skills and approaches are designed for the more formal kind of committee meeting. We would argue that it is precisely those informal encounters, working parties, *ad hoc* groups, loose discussion sessions, small group huddles and get togethers, that do need to work out a clear remit, negotiate as to available time and possible agenda and clarify roles and responsibilities. It is often argued that in these situations chairpersons are not necessary and that the group will organize itself. Certainly this does happen but even here it is quite a good idea to have someone keeping an eye on the time passing and the 'items' on the 'agenda' that remain to be discussed. We are really going back to some of the principles of time management (Chapter 3). Be assertive in setting your goals and helping others clarify theirs. The looser and friendlier the setting, the more this may be necessary and to everyone's eventual benefit.

Conclusion

The way in which a manager manages his or her team is of increasing importance in health and social care. Effective team work is a hallmark of effective management. Increasingly, through such devices as upward appraisal, managers are being judged (and rewarded) by the way their team is led and the individual members' perceptions of the effectiveness of this leadership.

References

Adair J (1986) *Effective Team Building*. Gower, Aldershot.
Belbin M (1981) *Managing Teams*. Heinemann, London.
Janis I L (1972) *Victims of Groupthink*. Houghton Mifflin, Boston.
Peters T (1992) *Liberation Management*. Macmillan, London.
Tuckman B (1965) *Development Sequence in Groups. Psychology Bulletin* 63,103–15.

Further reading

Burton G and Dimbleby R (1990) *Between Ourselves*. Edward Arnold, London.

7

The manager as conflict handler and negotiator

This chapter seeks to develop an increased understanding of the nature and sources of conflict and how we might handle it. We address an important approach to conflict handling, negotiation, as a positive and constructive way of bringing about a successful resolution for all concerned. We also examine aspects of problem solving and creative thinking that will help the manager to deal with situations that start in conflict but which, if managed well, can be turned into negotiation and problem solving.

Introduction

Conflict and disagreement are a normal and everyday part of organizational life. When we looked at team building in the last chapter, we mentioned that Belbin had found the need to introduce a role called 'plant' to the team in order to have someone who by nature was very willing to come up with new ideas and possibly create conflict by questioning the status quo.

Managers today reflect much about the need to manage in a context of rapid change. For some, change is an exciting prospect and many public service managers have experienced the last few years as amongst the most stimulating of their careers. On the other hand, the ability to manage change effectively has probably been the most testing challenge for all managers given the implications of change and the effects on all staff. In order to bring about change, we may have to 'destabilize' the existing order so that we can then begin to move people and the organization towards the new order that we consider to be desirable. It follows that this process of change, this search for innovation, for new and better ways of doing things involves a degree of conflict and disagreement within our own thinking as well as among our colleagues whom we are trying to manage.

Conflict and negotiation

Understanding the sources of conflict

The first step the manager has to undertake when dealing with conflict is to try to understand why it is happening. Generally speaking, people are in conflict or disagree because they hold legitimate points of view from their own perspectives. To begin with, an understanding of that perspective allows the disagreement to be 'managed'. One of the ways of doing this is to consider which of the following broad categories the source of conflict comes from:

- *Differences in values and principles.* For example the application of business thinking and the free market process to the public sector has been a major source of conflict. Professionals working in health care may feel that their principles in terms of delivery of health care to the individual patient are compromised by the process of looking at their activity from the point of view of marketing. On the plus side professionals have begun perhaps to identify the real added value they provide in their service.
- *Differences in perceptions.* A very common source of conflict is simply the situation where one person perceives a set of actions of another in a certain way which turns out to be unrelated to that person's original intention. In Chapter 4 we highlighted the importance of ensuring that the message sent by one person was clearly received, as intended, by the other.
- *Differences in expectations of outcomes.* We all know of situations where we may agree that some action is needed to solve a problem but do not agree about the most appropriate way to do it.
- *Unwillingness to negotiate or compromise.* Sometimes, managers have to deal with people who, for a variety of reasons, are unwilling to negotiate or shift from a position they take on some matter. These are often the most difficult situations for managers to deal with as there seems to be an almost unreasonable unwillingness to listen to reason.

Whatever the source of conflict, the important issue for the manager is to use questioning and listening techniques to get beneath the obviously stated position and find the *real* sources of disagreement. This allows the underlying interests or concerns which are 'feeding the conflict' to be brought to the surface and a beginning can be made to deal with them.

Once you have a clearer picture of the underlying reasons for the conflict there are a number of tactics that can be used to help manage it.

Resolving conflict

Differences in values and principles

Such differences as these are extreme and often the most difficult to resolve or reconcile. For example, if you believe in a divine origin and I do not, it is unlikely that we will change our positions, although our 'conflict' may lead to interesting debates. What usually happens in such circumstances is that we agree to differ. What is needed for us to continue to work together is a clear communication that although we may differ we still respect each other and are prepared to listen to the arguments. At a less extreme level the most useful tactic is to 'talk it out', i.e. to clarify where people stand. It is not unusual to find that people are nearer sharing fundamental values than they realize and the problem has been largely one of failure to listen and tolerate differences and failure to explain. If it is obvious, however, that so large a gap exists that attempting to resolve it is going to undermine the basis of a day-to-day working relationship, then it is probably best to avoid the confrontation.

Differences in perceptions

These can best be managed first of all through clear communication about how the different parties to a conflict actually perceive the situation. This in itself may be sufficient to resolve the conflict, as a frank and open exchange about how we all perceive the situation can actually lead to a wider perspective than each of the original positions. Secondly, we can seek to influence the other person's perception of the situation through, for example, presenting further evidence or through using selling techniques. Of course, you have to realize that the other party in the conflict may be trying to do exactly the same thing in relation to your perceptions of the situation.

Differences in expectations of outcomes

Here both parties agree that some action is needed to solve the problem, but do not agree about the best way to do it. A useful tactic, therefore, is to spend time brainstorming alternatives and turning the conflict into an exploration of these options with their various consequences. Quite often using this tactic, a 'third' alternative emerges as the best candidate and thus the conflict has been used to generate a novel way of dealing with the problem in a truly collaborative way.

Unwillingness to negotiate or compromise

If we find, as managers, that there are people who seem to be unreasonable and unprepared to 'listen to reason' then an ultimate tactic to resolving the conflict is for the manager to use positional power in the hierarchy to resolve the conflict and impose the solution. However, as we shall see later in looking at aspects of negotiation, an apparent unwillingness to negotiate may be a mask for underlying interests which need to be identified; so that indeed negotiation can take place around, on the one hand, how far these interests can be met, and, on the other hand, what you want in exchange for meeting these interests.

How to cope with conflict

In summary, as a manager there are probably only three options available to you to try to deal with conflict:

- Avoid the conflict, i.e. minimize the differences, perhaps procrastinate and avoid making decisions or simply deal with the symptoms rather than the causes.
- Square up or confront, i.e. do not give way, stick to your position: 'over my dead body!'
- Try to resolve the conflict.

In the short term you can perhaps make use of the first two to provide you with some thinking time or some breathing space, but realistically you eventually have to try to resolve the conflict. Such resolutions can involve negotiations and problem solving and the next sections of this chapter seek to address these approaches.

Negotiation

Negotiation in situations where conflict and disagreement is happening is probably the single most constructive approach that managers can take.

Negotiation can be defined as: 'the process of bargaining to reach a mutually acceptable agreement'.

A key feature worth emphasizing at this stage is that a negotiation can only take place if there is some basis for an 'exchange' – a bargain. If your senior manager asks 'Have you got a minute?' at a time when you have an urgent appointment with a client, the basis for an exchange is that the manager wants a bit of your time, perhaps to get your ideas about something or to brief you on some new work, and it appears that you are being given the opportunity to say where and when.

Kennedy (1992) has written and lectured widely on negotiating skills and helpfully suggests that there are essentially four key stages to any negotiation: *preparation, debate, proposition and closing.*

Preparation

Activities: setting your objectives, gathering information and determining your strategies.

Tactics:
- Set your objectives as follows: the *ideal*, i.e. the best you can hope to achieve, the *bottom line*, i.e. the least you would be prepared to settle for, and your *target*, i.e. what you are going to try for and perhaps have a realistic chance of achieving.
- Gather information not only to support your position but also in relation to what you think the other party wants to achieve and may be prepared

to offer. At this stage, your preparation is tentative because you may not be entirely clear what the other party's interests are.

Debate

Activities: encouraging the other party to determine what they are interested in and revealing your own initial bargaining position. Exploring the problem.

Tactics:
- Make use of listening and questioning at this stage to help to assess and discover the other party's objectives and requirements, what they want and what they are prepared to concede.
- Assess the other party's strengths and weaknesses in their case and observe their tactics in the negotiating situation.
- Try to get beneath the stances as presented to the underlying interests, e.g. the values underlying the position being presented.

Proposition

Activity: bargaining or trading to find common ground involving the willingness of the other party to move and revealing your willingness to concede in some areas.

Tactics:
- Use conditional propositions of the form 'if I do this will you consider doing that?'
- Never make one-sided concessions, always seek to link a concession on your part with a concession on the other person's part that you want.
- 'Nothing is agreed until everything is agreed', thus if possible, negotiate the whole package rather than agree parts in a piecemeal fashion. This avoids the problem of hidden agenda, where a major concession is suddenly requested.
- Be aware of the importance of 'signalling'. This is the technique that people use to say one thing but actually to give an indication that they mean something slightly different. For example 'This is what we normally do...' is the signal for 'We are willing to discuss some variation from what we usually do'.

Closing

Activity: arriving at the final position which, of course, may include 'no deal' if the 'price is too high'. Entering into an agreement which may take a written, contractual form or simply an exchange of memos summarizing what has been agreed.

Tactics:

- Use summarizing to emphasize the concessions made and the areas of agreement arrived at so far.
- Be prepared to offer minor concessions in return for agreement to settle.
- Complete the agreement, perhaps by such simple methods as splitting the difference in some contentious but relatively minor area.

Knowing which stage you are at in any negotiation helps to determine the types of tactics you might use and the particular skills which are necessary at each of these four stages. The preparation stage in particular is worth investment of time. As a rule of thumb, it is worth spending as much time in preparation as you think the negotiation itself is going to take. Most negotiations go through these various stages although there may be a degree of moving backwards and forwards from one stage to another.

Some other useful comments on negotiations are the following:

- *Nothing is agreed until everything is agreed!* Although you may be negotiating details and agreeing elements as you go along, remember that until everything is agreed all aspects are open to renegotiation. Thus *all aspects of an agreement are interlinked.*
- *If you don't ask, you don't get!* Always start with the assumption that everything is negotiable. Do not talk or think yourself out of a possibility – be optimistic.
- *Negotiations are about adding value – your gain and their gain.* Let the negotiation become a search for the added values for yourself and for the other party. Satisfying each other's added values goes a long way to achieving a successful conclusion.

The skills of negotiation

A range of skills can be identified as being important in negotiations. It is quite likely that no one person would be competent in all aspects of this and it therefore follows that in many negotiating situations it is desirable for small teams of two or three people to be set up in order to ensure that the range of skills needed are represented in the team.

The range of skills used in negotiation can be summarized as the abilities to:

- analyse and assess information;
- identify objectives - the 'must haves' and the 'would like to haves';
- prepare arguments and proposals;
- communicate, particularly questioning and listening;
- present a case, particularly oral presentations;
- debate, i.e. to respond to ideas and proposals 'off the top of your head';
- control the meeting and particularly to control speakers; and

- ensure the summarizing of progress, clarifying the situation and conclud-
  ing agreements – chairing skills.

Activity

Consider the following questions. What are your strengths? What are
your weaknesses? Can you bring in a colleague to strengthen your
negotiating approach?

Styles of negotiation

Take a look at Case study 7.1.

Case study 7.1

Imagine the situation – it is about 10.00 pm in a busy city restaurant on
a Saturday night. It has been a fraught evening and tempers are a bit
short. The two participants in our drama – the chef and his assistant –
both need a lemon to complete a dish they are working on but unfortunately there is only one left. Both chefs grab for it and an argument
breaks out - eventually the head-chef pulls rank and uses it for his dish,
leaving his junior to do what he can without one. However, if they had
stopped for a moment to explain and discuss what they wanted a lemon
for, they would have discovered that the one needed the peel to
complete a sauce and the other needed the juice to finish off a sweet
dish. There was potential for both succeeding in their objectives but
unwillingness to discuss and listen to each other created the problem.

When people are observed in negotiating situations they often adopt one of
two different styles of negotiating:

Hard positional – sometimes called 'tough guy' and characterized by:

- wanting to win
- viewing the other person or party as an adversary
- seeing the negotiation as a contest of wills, a bit like a chess game
- taking particular positions over issues and hanging on to them.

Soft positional – sometimes called 'tender guy' and characterized by:

- wanting to avoid conflict and make friends
- conceding generously and changing positions fairly easily
- backing down when threatened
- avoiding a contest of wills.

A problem-solving approach

A problem-solving approach to negotiation is a third and, in our view, a more appropriate way to seek to resolve differences. In summary, this approach is characterized by:

- Approaching the negotiation as a partnership often between profession-als who have the common concern to identify and solve problems. The assumption here is that both parties wish to find a solution. It is akin to the adult-to-adult ego state as discussed in Chapter 4.
- Focusing on the interests and values underlying the conflict rather than the positions and stances taken by individuals. The negotiation thus becomes a search to find the real underlying interests of both parties rather than an opportunity to score points.
- Seeing the negotiation as a process of inventing options to solve the problems as identified, rather than as an opportunity to 'get my own way'. The process of seeking options draws on our ability to think in a creative way and will be discussed more fully later.
- Seeking agreement about the standards to be used to determine fair outcomes rather than relying on matters of opinion or strengths of personality. Typical negotiations with external contractors on such details as the length of time for payment after submission of invoice can often be agreed on the basis of what is a standard in the industry.
- In the preparation phase of a negotiation, it is wise to consider what the alternative may be if an agreement is not possible, i.e. what will you do if you do not have a deal? The reasoning behind this is that by careful consideration of what your alternatives are, you increase your confidence during the negotiating process itself. Clearly, if you go into a negotiation feeling that you *have* to conclude an agreement of some kind, then this is quickly detected by the other party and can be exploited as a weakness.

Activity

Think through these different styles and reflect on a recent negotiation that you have been involved in. What was your preferred style? Do you think you could move more towards a problem-solving approach? What aspects of your style do you need to work on to move in this direction?

Creative thinking and problem solving

At various stages in a negotiation of a problem-solving type, we have seen the importance of creative thinking. Some of the typical barriers to creative thinking are the following.

- Allowing your mind to become fixed in a particular way of thinking about a situation or problem: 'I did it this way last time so I will do it this way again!'
- Not identifying and possibly challenging the underlying assumptions we make and thus preventing new ways of looking at the situation. How often have we heard the statement 'We can't possibly afford to do that!'
- Being conditioned to think mainly in sequential A. B. C. D... steps – sometimes called vertical or logical thinking, rather than using lateral ways of thinking.
- Being afraid of looking stupid.
- Evaluating too quickly – subjecting a very new idea to highly critical thinking too early and before it has been given a chance to germinate and develop. At meetings, for example, there is usually someone who is very willing to 'shoot down' a new idea almost as soon as it has appeared.
- Tending to polarize alternatives into this or that possibilities instead of considering many possibilities.

Activity

Consider the following problem. You are sitting a physics examination and the question you are tackling is: 'Given a barometer, how would you measure the height of a building?'
Take a moment to think of ways of handling this question.
We will return to it in a moment.

Generally, all these barriers revolve around the concept of 'mindsets' – these are stereotyped ways in which you perceive and approach problems. In negotiations, mindsets can lead us to view a situation from one particular perspective – the right one of course – and may prevent us from exploring alternatives.

The main way of coping with mindsets is to challenge the assumptions and be prepared, however humble this may appear, to accept that you may be wrong or that there may be another way of looking at something. In a team setting, you can make use of the person who is good at thinking in this way.

So, going back to the barometer question, what did you come up with? Many people would rack their brains to remember how a barometer works and the formula for calculating pressure change in relation to height. Something like: 'I would measure the pressure at the bottom of the building and again at the top and by some formula work out the height that way!'

That is certainly one way of solving the problem and, for some, it may be viewed as the 'right' way because you are sitting a physics exam and this is a physics-type answer.

But perhaps you also realized that it was by no means the only way to look at the problem provided that you can challenge the assumption that a physics-type answer must be given. For example you might have thought of some of the following:

- Get a long piece of string, tie the barometer to one end and dangle it over the edge of the building and then measure the string. The problem does not necessarily preclude the use of other bits and pieces.
- Go to the top of the building and drop the barometer off the edge and time how long it takes to hit the ground. There is a formula for determining the rate of acceleration which will give the distance as well. Note there is nothing to suggest that the barometer has to be intact at the end of the experiment.
- You happen to know that the caretaker in the building is a keen collector of antiques. You can go to him and in return for the barometer get him to tell you the height of the building.
- Measure the length of the barometer and then use it as a ruler to measure the internal wall of one floor and then multiply this by the total number of floors. In this solution, you see the barometer as a measure of something other than only pressure.

So is there a right answer? We would suggest that there is an appropriate or optimum solution depending on a range of factors. For example, having generated many possible solutions (and you may have thought of many more) you would then apply criteria to evaluate these. Such criteria might include: cost, speed, ease of solution, accuracy, and so on, and by systematically applying these you can identify the optimum solution. For example, the caretaker is likely to give the most accurate answer, but at a cost, whereas the use of string is probably the easiest and cheapest although a little time consuming.

Edward de Bono (1985) has offered us a useful insight into different modes of thinking which may help in this creative thinking process. He summarises his approach with reference to 'six thinking hats', each of which emphasizes a different kind of thinking, and all of which are valuable at some point in trying to analyse and solve problems. These six hats are assigned different colours and are as follows:

- *Red hat thinking:* Wearing the red hat encourages the thinker to express how they feel about something, e.g. ordinary emotions like fear, dislike and suspicion and the more complex feelings in making judgements such as the well-known nurse's 'intuition' or the manager's 'hunch'.
- *Blue hat thinking:* This thinking involves organizing the thinking process, defining problems and shaping questions. With your blue hat on, you think of summaries and conclusions, monitor progress and ensure that rules are followed.
- *White hat thinking:* This thinking deals in facts and figures, is logical and objective. It is neutral, offers no interpretations or opinions and is disciplined in approach.

- *Yellow hat thinking:* This thinking is positive, constructive, optimistic and concerned with making things happen. There is a search here for values and benefits and a seeking out of opportunities to exploit them.
- *Green hat thinking:* This is the creative hat. The colour symbolizes the fertility and growth of seeds or ideas. The fundamental aspect of green hat thinking is the search for alternatives. It is this thinking hat which is most powerful in challenging the mindsets.
- *Black hat thinking:* The black hat thinker points out what is wrong, why things will not work, what the risks are and what the dangers are. It is a devil's advocate hat. In a more positive sense it is the source of evaluation and constructive and critical thinking. Although creative thinkers often find black hat thinking destructive, in practice it can also be a source of challenging mindsets, i.e. that it is critical of stereotyped approaches to problems.

In dealing with conflict, using a problem-solving negotiating style, the explicit use of the different thinking hats can be of particular value at various stages. For example, in the preparation phase yellow hat thinking is optimistic and helps to search for underlying values and interests; at the debating stage, red hat thinking permits access to feelings about suggestions that are being made; at the proposition stage, green hat thinking allows full exploration of alternatives; with white hat thinking, cool and logical assessments take place; and at the closing stage yellow hat and black hat thinking combine optimism with a critical evaluation of the agreement that is being arrived at.

Conclusion

Negotiation is concerned with problem solving. It is not something that is reserved for senior managers. We can all use these aspects of negotiation to assist us with solving problems at work. Remember, the crucial aspect is that 'both sides can and should win'. We should abandon the notion that negotiation is about doing down the other party; it is essentially concerned with solving problems and healing differences. That is why creative thinking can be so helpful in finding ways to unknot the tangles that we face in our dealings with colleagues, bosses and patients.

References

De Bono E (1985) *Six Thinking Hats*. Penguin Books, Harmondsworth.
Kennedy G (1992) *The Perfect Negotiation. All you need to get it right first time.* Century Business, London.

Further reading

Fisher R and Ury W (1988) *Getting to Yes: negotiating for agreement without giving in.* Houghton Mifflin, Boston.

Freund J C (1992) *Smart Negotiation: How to make deals in the real world.* Simon & Schuster, New York.

8

The manager of communications

In this chapter we deal with the role of manager as responsible for seeing that internal communications are in good working order. We look at some of the criteria for successful internal communications and examine a case study where despite the manager's enthusiasm for communications there was a failure to plan the resources necessary. We also provide some advice for the management of external communications.

Introduction

In Chapter 4 we examined some of the ingredients necessary for the manager to communicate successfully with staff, colleagues, patients and clients. Now we change the focus to the manager organising, evaluating and assisting the communication process throughout the workplace. Most textbooks on management feature communications skills and how essential it is for all managers to possess them; not so many comment on the skills the manager should possess in actually managing communications in the workplace.

Surveys of organizations and readings of the *Health Service Journal* and *Nursing Times* over the last few years suggest that the quality of the communication flow between members of staff is of fundamental importance to the success of the organization. We should not be too surprised at this: any organization needs to be able to keep its members informed of where it is going, which directions it proposes to take and who will be playing what part in the journey. This is particularly important during a time of rapid change. We have seen that for management of change to be carried through well requires effective communication to all staff. You may have worked in an organization where staff morale was lowered by feelings of uncertainty as to where the management was taking the staff. You may have felt that you had not even been given a sight of the map, never mind joined in the walk.

Despite the fact that the quality of communication between staff in any organization is crucial, managers often ignore it unless something goes wrong. The assumption that all is well unless there is a breakdown can partially be attributed to inertia as well as a feeling that 'if it ain't broke don't fix it'. This can be countered by pointing out that if everything has gone quiet then perhaps the engine has stopped.

Effective listening and good presentation and good interview skills were just some of the ingredients needed by managers to be successful communicators. When it comes to the management of communications we suggest from our work in conducting reviews of communication in hospitals and health boards and from similar surveys, that the criteria discussed below are important.

Criteria for managing communications

Reliability

The consumers of the communication – the users – need to feel that they can rely on the information contained in the memos, notices, letters, reports, public pronouncements, e-mail, staff newsletters, etc. that come from management. Credibility is such a precious commodity: it takes a long time to build up but it can seep away quickly. There is little point in having a very elaborate (often expensive) system of getting information to all staff if at the end they do not believe the truth of what they being told. The message received is only as good as the message given.

We have seen in Chapter 4 that the receivers' attitudes to the intended communication play a large role as to whether they will accept the information or not. It is essential to ensure that the mechanism of communication is as reliable as possible. This is why it is important to establish and monitor procedures and to set standards.

Bad news is never pleasant or easy to accept. Indications from audits suggest that if the manager comes and talks directly to those affected face to face, the pain is a little easier to accept. This acceptance, often reluctant and in many cases only partial, depends greatly on the way that the information is transmitted.

Credibility of managers' communication

What tends to reduce managers' credibility is when there is a delay in passing the news on and then only some of it is released, in dribs and drabs, or when a representative of the manager is wheeled in to pour oil on troubled waters.

We came across an example of delay from a communications survey in a hospital where a member of the nursing staff found out that her ward was to close. She heard about it from someone on the bus as she was travelling home from work. You can imagine what that kind of information does to the credibility of managers running the system. At this point some of you will say: 'well that's the typical rumour mill working, we can't control that'. We would counter this by saying that all organizations have their unofficial sources of communication such as the grapevine. However, where there tends to be a lack, a delay or loss of credibility in official communication then any such rumour mill will grind away overtime to fill in the gaps. This should not surprise us. The more anxiety staff have about what is happening the more that grapevine will be used. In these situations, when we are in the dark, we need light.

Notice we said that managers should come and talk to staff. We cannot emphasize this enough. In a June 1994 address the Secretary of State for Health in the UK said that more Trust managers should spend less of their time talking about mission statements and more time actually talking to the staff and sharing ideas with them.

Importance of face-to-face communication

In the private sector, a survey of staff at the Royal Bank of Scotland under-taken in 1993 showed overwhelmingly that half the staff got most of their information from circulars, whereas what they wanted was communication from the boss, face to face. We have already recommended MBWA (manag-ing by walking about) in Chapter 4. Sending a memo or an emissary is one thing, but these cannot replace face-to-face contact. It takes a certain kind of moral courage to come and confront staff with bad news. Flak (and fur) may fly and uncomfortable words be expressed. However it is much better that this should happen and be dealt with on the spot, rather than be allowed to fester and create all kinds of bad feeling and disappointment.

In times of rapid change in health and social care management, it is even more important to make sure that information flow to all staff is rapid and personalized. It appears to us that it is precisely at these times when staff are really hungry for information, that the news channels tend to dry up and a freeze occurs. If a manager can respond to staff's need for news and give a frank account as far as he or she knows of the situation, some but not all staff will listen and the manager's credibility will possibly remain unaffected, even enhanced. ('Well she did have the bottle to tell us straight.') In some cases managers may not themselves know much more than their staff, as the decision is to be made over their heads. This is no excuse, we suggest, for any delay: even if one does not have the complete picture, staff need to know what is known and what is not known.

Confidentiality

That brings us to the thorny issue of confidentiality. We suggest that organi-zations deliberately review what aspects of their work should be classified as confidential.

The exceptions would be staff personnel files and information relating to particularly sensitive commercial/contractual information. Are managers in the health and social care services perhaps too keen to reach for the CONFIDENTIAL stamp? Have you and your management colleagues reviewed your criteria for imposing a confidential embargo on what could be news and information for your staff? Do you ever make use of 'confidentiality' as an excuse to create a barrier between yourself, other managers and staff?

We suggest that people who work with you will, on the whole, understand that some files cannot be revealed, but your credibility and therefore the reliability of the communication you send out may be enhanced by a display of openness. There may be a particular problem in health and social care regarding confidentiality as all staff are naturally very conscious of the interests of their patients and the issues that now constrain everyone under the provisions of the Data Protection Act 1984 (*see* page 188).

Reaching parts that others can't!

Does the communication actually reach those parts it is supposed to? We have come across many examples where managers were confident that the communication was getting down through the organization, only to be surprised when the evidence was presented to them that it had, in fact, got stuck.

Problems of communicating outside the core

There is a growing tendency within health and social care for the 'core staff' to become smaller and smaller and for more and more part timers to be taken on. This poses a very real problem for managers in trying to communicate adequately with all staff. In the UK over the last few years many services within hospitals have been contracted out and in some cases outside companies have won the tender. This process, the development of a shrinking core and the extended numbers of part time/contracted out staff, has placed new demands on managers to make sure that their communication does in fact reach to all parts.

In some cases staff of the outside company will not see that they have any responsibility to communicate with or receive communication from the 'host' organization. This can be a very real problem when it comes to their staff attending your meetings. It is an issue some authorities have faced up to by insisting that certain meetings and lines of communication are established and expected as part of the terms of the contract. This is where standards, long since part and parcel of contracts when it comes to standards of health and hygiene, should be extended to expectations of communication.

How do I know if the message is getting through?

To test the way in which your communication is penetrating the ranks of part time, night shift and contracted out service staff, you would be advised to do some practical testing. When you have sent out a notice to all staff, try telephoning various people at various points in the communication chain. Do this at differently spaced time intervals so that you will be able to see who receives what and when.

You may be surprised. Some slowness in the system may be because of physical layout difficulties of the site you are working with, the arrangement of offices and the spaces between for the internal mail to cover. Many of these problems can be tackled through discussions with administration staff and those running the internal postal service. You should, while undertaking such a review, consider the whole issue of standards, as mentioned earlier. Standards here will refer to expected pick up and delivery times between sites, what constitutes urgent mail and how this is to be delivered, etc.

The same kind of review can be achieved with the issue of notices, team briefings, etc. One practical idea is to use colour coding for mail deliveries; this will enable each site/department to be more rapidly identified by the mail room, porters and others who do the actual distribution. This system of colour coding can also be used to designate priority.

Some of the problem in passing information down the line ties in with our comments in Chapter 4 on attitudes and their effects on communication. We saw there how we tend to pay attention to things that are in line with our attitudinal position and ignore, select out or discount those which fall outside these parameters. This will help to explain why some people in the chain of communication do not pass material on, or if they do it is in a very selected and distorted form.

Team briefing

Some organizations have experimented with team briefing systems. We examined these briefly earlier. The theory is that from the time the senior manager has announced the core brief to the time when the most junior members of staff have heard the core and the local brief no more than 24 or 36 hours will have elapsed even with very large organizations.

The aim behind team briefing is thus to ensure that there is a rapid, reliable and penetrative system of communication. In our experience and from talking to those who have tried this system, we have to admit that in health and social care establishments there are severe problems that mitigate against its success. The first of these is that, unlike many private organizations that have put team briefing into place, there are large numbers of staff in health and social care who are part time, shift employees and, increasingly within the UK, contracted out staff. This has made the operation of the system difficult. Secondly, in some cases known to us, insufficient attention has been given to adapting the system from its source, often the Industrial Society, to the peculiar needs of the hospital, social care agency, etc.

Thirdly, we suspect that in some cases the system has not been given enough time to settle in and find its feet. There has not been enough training and support given to the staff involved before the system is disbanded.

Activity

What do you feel should be the criteria for the success of any team briefing system? Jot them down before you read further.

Criteria for a successful team briefing system could include the following.

- The whole staff group should be involved in the planning, formation, review and adaptation where necessary of the system. Too often team briefing is instituted as a *fait accompli*. If we really believe in the empowerment of staff then this is precisely where discussions have to be held and opinions and objections listened to.
- The system should be planned and presented not just as a one way operation where bosses tell staff, but as a two way channel which provides opportunities for staff to inform the briefer of their concerns and raise questions that they know will be answered. Managers should be very careful to adhere to promises regarding the speedy return of answers to staff questions and enquiries. (To be fair to the Industrial Society and to many of the team briefing schemes 'on the market', the intention was to encourage upward communication.)
- With large institutions it may be a good idea to pilot a team briefing system within one section so as to get some grip on the likely problems. Such pilots should allow the system to become more tuned to the needs of the particular hospital, health board or social care establishment. For instance, the development of Clinical Directorates within many NHS hospitals will enable some kind of modified team briefing to be developed.
- Resources must be put into the system: this means training the briefers, supporting their progress, spending time with part time and night staff to see if their needs are being taken into consideration. We do know of centres where an adapted and specially modified form of team briefing is working with the general support of the staff and where the upward flow of communication has become almost as important as the downward.

QUICK and stakeholders meetings

WEB Associates have recommended to organizations a variation on the team briefing system. This is entitled the QUICK meeting: Questioning, Understanding, Informing, Challenging, Knowing.

The system works as follows: a group of named people (not necessarily the head of department or team leaders) are designated who can be called at very short notice to meet with the senior manager. They are presented with the information and vested with the authority to pass this on to a particular group of staff. Attendance at such meetings is mandatory. The important aspect is that the system must be able to work rapidly. It is used only for important news which affects all staff. It seeks to prevent the all too frequent occurrence where staff find out what is happening to their establishment from their local or national newspapers.

We also recommend 'stakeholders' meetings, which all staff are eligible to attend, as are shareholders in a public limited company. These should be held at least annually or when there is some important strategy to announce. Because of the nature of the shift patterns worked by staff, in reality this means that senior managers will have to hold a number of such meetings during a period of 24 hours.

The development of new technology: e-mail, fax, mobile phones, video conferencing, etc.– offers various possibilities for managers to keep in touch with staff and for staff to keep in touch with them. These developments are likely to be welcomed particularly with those staff in outlying and remote areas, operating at nights and weekends. However, despite these advances we are confident that nothing will replace the importance of face-to-face contact.

Perseverance

We have already mentioned that some communication systems are put into place and then abandoned. This can have damaging effects on managers' credibility and the likely success of other initiatives. Some of this may be due to senior managers being on short term contracts and their desire to make a name for themselves in that time by instituting something spectacular or abandoning something in an equally spectacular fashion.

Sometimes the abandonment occurs because there is a shift in priorities or revenue allocation. Whatever the cause we would recommend that managers should be slow to cancel an initiative in communication unless there is overwhelming evidence that it is not working and staff morale and efficiency is suffering. It is often far better to review it and generally adapt it to your special needs than to let it die without trace and have staff wag their heads and say, 'Another waste of time and money. I wonder what they will dream up next'.

Understandability

The *Sunday Times* Insight Team carried out a survey of management–staff communications at the late British Leyland Company during the early 1970s. It examined principally the readability of the memos that were sent to staff. They interviewed staff who had read the memos and found that many of them only remembered the 'Happy Christmas' or 'Best Wishes' at the end. The average length of sentence in the memos studied was thirty-five words.

Here an example from a very urgent and important memo sent out to all staff:

> The managing director has made it clear to all Plant Committees that neither he nor his directors will be submitting any major capital expenditure for final approval to either the British Leyland Board or the National Enterprise Board unless he has commitments to the necessary improvements in productivity from employees representatives of all sections and all management involved in the respective project.

The question behind this episode for you as managers is: Are you operating like British Leyland's memo writers? Do your staff and colleagues understand fully what you write to them? Have you ever tested your written communication for its readability? Would your work pass the Plain English Society's approval or would you be awarded one of their prizes for gobble-dygook?

In an article in the *Financial Times* (3 June 1994), Simon Gibson was bemoaning the current trend for bosses to resort to management-speak rather than use clear and original expression. He pin-pointed the increasing use of jargon – words such as downsizing, proactive, networking, etc. which have been borrowed from computing and are now applied willy nilly to all kinds of management edicts. Even phrases such as 'total quality management' he suggests have become so often used that they are in danger of becoming meaningless. Jargon is a useful short cut between those who understand what it is all about. When it is used between such people then there can be no complaint. There are problems if it is used when the level of understanding of one of the parties is lacking, and unless there is an explanation provided that party may be seriously disadvantaged.

A further aspect of understandability is that many staff are sent masses of information and huge quantities of paper. We would recommend that reports should be summarized and much of this paper mountain reduced to abstracts that are then sent out to all staff. Those interested in looking at the complete version can ask for it or read it at some central point or library.

Tone

'It's not what you say, it's the way that you say it'. Sometimes we produce communication with staff which is free of jargon, plain and direct but still fails to hit the mark in that staff do not pay attention. We briefly touched on the main parameters of Transactional Analysis in Chapter 4 and examined some of the problems when communication takes place from the 'parent' state and how it can easily trigger off the 'child' response.

Consider the tone of the memos and notices you send out. Consider the tone of your presentations to staff and colleagues. Think back to the last report you gave to a committee of management. How do you think your readers and listeners felt about the tone of what you communicated? Does it appear to your listeners that they are being scolded?

As we said in the review of Transactional Analysis, the tone of what is communicated can influence the climate of the organization we work in. If managers write the following kind of memo to staff (spotted on a staff noticeboard) then the climate is likely to be rather frosty and any notion of empowerment will be taken at face value only.

> I remind you all, yet again, not to leave any sharp objects in uniform pockets. Such downright carelessness causes considerable nuisance and risk to laundry staff. Let this be the last time I have to take the time and trouble to notify you.

Activity

How could this be rephrased on a more adult to adult tone ? How could the parent–child be made more neutral? Try your hand at a rewrite and then have a look at this one below.

> Staff in the laundry are experiencing very real problems with sharp objects such as scissors and nail files which have been left in the pockets of your uniforms when sent for cleaning. A previous memo doesn't appear to have done the trick so I am asking you again. We have had two cases of laundry staff receiving injuries as a result of handling sharp objects.
> Please make it a habit to check all pockets before someone gets really hurt.

Do you feel this carries the information and is now acceptable in tone?

Activity

Read Case study 8.1. What advice would you give to the directors and their senior management team?

Case study 8.1

The Chief Executive of XY Social Care Agency has for some time felt unhappy with the communication amongst staff. He is determined to take action. He puts the idea of a monthly staff bulletin to his senior management team at their monthly meeting. He has seen such bulletins in use in similar organizations and feels that such a vehicle would do wonders for interstaff communication.

The senior management team are equally keen to see improvements; they are aware that many staff appear to be left behind in the news stakes; there have been complaints about people being bypassed and a favoured few getting the news before the others. They, as a team, are pleased that their director wants to do something; they have been advocating a review of existing interstaff communication for some time but with no success. Their director is well known for his enthusiasms and it is always important to exploit them quickly before his attention moves to something else. At the meeting several of the team expressed their concern as to resources and personnel being committed to such a venture.

The director assured the team that he would personally find the resources for at least the first two issues; he would make use of his personal assistant and some of the admin staff. The important thing, according to the director, was to get the project off the ground. He asked at this meeting for any important news from the members of the team to go into the first bulletin.

The first issue is indeed produced to deadline, mainly as a result of the director and his PA working very hard on it. (He even takes home his laptop computer and spends several evenings on it, finishing it at about midnight on the night before the deadline for printing.) During the days which follow the first issue staff appear to find that it has been a useful venture although several say what a pity they were not informed about it earlier then they could have made some contribution. However it soon becomes apparent that there are staff who have not received a copy for some reason or another. At the senior management meeting following the launch of the bulletin several managers asked about future policy. The director said that as he had got the first issue out on time he would be expecting his managers to take more responsibility for subsequent issues. This idea was not well received. The director then said that he would make the time to produce number two with one of the managers and that he was looking for a volunteer. Under his gaze one of the team 'steps forward' and the plan and deadline is agreed.

Three months later in the canteen a member of staff says to her colleague 'What happened to the staff bulletin? It seemed a good idea at the time especially for someone like me who only works part time. I only remember seeing one edition'. Her colleague replies,'Well, you're lucky I've never even seen a copy; there was some reference to it at our staff meeting. In fact our manager asked us if we could form a group to take over the production of a regular staff bulletin. We told her, she must be joking!'

Your advice may have included the following.

- *Failure to plan*. Any initiative such as this requires planning. This is one of the primary duties of the manager (think of PIE from Chapter 2). For all his obvious enthusiasm there is no way that such a scheme as this should be launched in such a manner. We can see what happens as a result: once the personal enthusiasm evaporates or is lost to other projects so it tends to be handed on, or dropped down, on to the laps of other colleagues. Inevitably we get the dwindling effect: what was once a promising project declines with all the consequent effects on staff morale. It was all very fine for the manager to get the project up and running (assuming there had been sufficient consultation with his colleagues) but for him to spend evenings typing away may not have been the most *effective* use of his time. Remember this important distinction between effective and efficient.

- *Effective management.* This director may have been a very efficient user of his laptop and performed well in putting the bulletin together but we may well comment on whether this was an effective use of his time, given his salary and responsibilities. It might have been more effective if he had planned a strategy for the bulletin, considered the available resources, set in motion some proper distribution system and harnessed the enthusiasm and energy of staff who would be more efficient than him.

Strategies

Many organizations have developed and are developing communication strategies. These are the route maps which should guide the organization and set out standards expected in the way communication is handled.

The 1994 UK Audit Commission's report *Trusting in the Future* identified poor communication as one of the factors contributing to variable performance in NHS Trusts. The Commission reported that half of those Trusts they investigated had some communication strategy. The main objectives for internal communication were:

- making sure that all staff understood the main aims of the organizations;
- encouraging team work and a sense of corporateness, consulting all staff; and
- keeping them up to date on developments and being receptive to ideas and comments from all staff.

There is, of course, all the difference between having a communication strategy nicely framed on the staff noticeboards and the reality of what actually happens.

Do you have a communications strategy? Have you ever reviewed communications in your place of work to find out what staff think about communications, where they feel improvements could be made, what ideas they have for coping with the needs of staff who work on shifts? Have you ever considered the nature of upward communications from staff to managers? Is there a suggestion scheme and if so does it work? Does it have the trust of staff? Are there improvements to be made?

Carrying out a review or audit of communications is not all about finding out bad news, the holes in the system, the negative, it is also about discovering and confirming where the successes are, the positive aspects of communication so that these can be built on and developed.

Audits of communication

As with any survey, review or audit (the name is different but the process is essentially the same – some managers consider 'audit' to be too full of negative connotations and use the more neutral 'survey'), it is important to plan the operation carefully. Is it to be a whole staff survey or are you just going to concentrate on one department, or on one aspect such as the working of the internal mail system?

We would certainly urge you from the start of your planning to take the staff fully into your thinking and work out how the information is to be released to them following the completion of the survey. The Royal Bank of Scotland survey referred to earlier revealed that 63 per cent of staff surveyed said that the results of the previous survey had not even been discussed with them by their bosses. As the article in *The Scotsman* concluded: 'What is the point of an exercise like this, opening up the promise of consultation and of more local and individual concerns being addressed when the middle and junior management simply shoves it in the "pending" tray and forgets it.'

So whatever you do, make sure *the results* are discussed with all staff and if possible try to find something to act on as a result of the audit. Far too often the audit comes and goes, the answers to the interviews and questionnaires are forgotten and nothing appears to change. Staff quite rightly say: 'What was all that fuss about then? Things just stay the same.'

Our advice is to get something done as a result of the audit: it may only be a small thing such as the re-siting and enlargement of a noticeboard but it will send out the right signals.

It is important to keep the momentum for change going. Here you might like to think of your communications strategy and see the audit as forming part of that.

One aspect that any audit will throw up is the skills level of staff in communications. Part of your strategy will be to explore the need for specific training of staff: in chairing meetings, making presentations, writing abstracts of reports, effective letter writing, telephone, reception and customer care skills, etc.

Appointment of communications officer

You might also consider whether it would be useful to have one member of your staff designated as the communications person. There are obvious dangers here in that people will assume that he or she will do all that is necessary and in double quick time, and therefore not bother overmuch themselves. However, it might be useful to have this one person (it might only be a part of the job) to take on board responsibility for coordinating and managing communications within the unit/department/office etc. This will not mean that you as manager will be able to duck out of this responsibility but there will be a named person whom staff can approach, who can hold meetings, initiate surveys, oversee a staff bulletin, monitor the noticeboards, etc. Because of the lack of space, we refer you to texts that cover such audits. We would urge you to think about some of the various techniques that you might use when conducting the audit.

In Chapter 13 we cover some of these techniques, such as interviewing, the development and testing of questionnaires, observation and shadowing which are useful in carrying out any audit.

External communication

We have been concerned so far with the manager's responsibilities for internal communication. However the manager must also be aware and plan for the demands of external communication. This will involve getting the corporate message across to the community, to the media and to various targeted individuals – opinion formers. This is a vast subject in itself and large organizations normally have some PR or external affairs person who has responsibility for this.

Handling the media

Let us suppose that you do not have such a person on your staff and that the local press phones you up with a demand for information – is it true that a large number of your staff are going to be made redundant? What is your reaction? Have you prepared yourself for this?

So we return to the importance – the absolute necessity of planning. It is often a terrible mistake to speak off the cuff to the media. External communications have to be planned for in just the same way as internal communications. You need a policy. You need to nominate people who can do the job; you need to set standards and create expectations.

You also need to take seriously the issue of training. You cannot expect staff to handle press releases and conduct interviews with the media unless they have had some training. This does not come cheap since you usually need to be coached by media professionals. The expense can be justified when you consider the potentially damaging consequences to you, your staff and the whole organization of giving the wrong impression to the community. You probably have your own horror story of the time when a manager said the wrong thing to the press and had to be contradicted by someone higher up, the damage already having been done to staff morale.

We would advise you as manager to carry out some disaster planning when it comes to external communications. What plans have you for that special situation? How would you and your staff handle inquiries if a patient...? if one of your staff...? Naturally as with all disaster planning, one cannot rehearse all the scenarios that may happen but such planning does get one into the way of proactive rather than merely reactive thinking and responses.

Activity

Read the following questions and think how you would react to them before you read further.

A If you were away and something happened in your section and the press called who would answer for you?
B If your local radio station called you up for an interview on your future plans for care in the community, and only gave you a morning's notice what would you do?
C If one of your staff wrote a letter to the local paper criticizing the way you and your management colleagues were cutting staff, what would you do?

A.   This is precisely the kind of situation where training and role clarification are essential. Just imagine the consequences if there is a delay in making a response to some controversial news. We have discussed delegation at some length in Chapter 2. This is a good example of a situation in which planned delegation is essential; the person nominated to speak for you must be coached and supported and not expected to be able to jump right in.

B.   The nature of the media and the nature of news is that much of it is unexpected and calls for interviews can come out of the blue. Remember, however, what we said in Chapter 3 on time management. Unexpected events can, if analysed, often fall into a pattern and can be 'planned' for. We recommend you find out the names of those journalists concerned with health and social care matters; get to know them; invite them in to see your work. This way you will probably have an opportunity to get into their thinking, and the unexpected phone call can be that much less unexpected. Cultivate your media contacts and they will help you. Tell them what stories you have coming up – new developments, interesting human interest angles. Involve your staff in media awareness so that it is not just you and your management colleagues hobnobbing with the media but a whole staff effort to see their work more widely noticed and appreciated.

  Learn how to produce crisp, concise press releases and if you have gained good contacts with journalists, both newspapers, radio and TV, then most if not all your material will be used. Remember that journalists always are looking for news and try to satisfy that hunger.

C.   Quick reaction needed here. Delay implies lack of certainty as to one's position. Not to reply is seldom wise. The damage has already been done. Criticisms need to be answered. There are very few occasions when to stay silent in the face of criticism is the better policy. If staff have to go to these lengths it usually says something about the climate of trust within the organization and the communications procedures that are in place to answer individual criticisms. Much has been made about the problem of 'whistle-blowers', those staff who wish to make a complaint about some aspect of their work but who fear reprisal from managers if they do. If staff have to go to the press to give vent to their feelings then that says something about the climate of trust and the effectiveness of upward communication systems in place. Having responded to the criticism, then it is time to tackle the issues which produced the explosion.

We would urge all managers to take these matters very seriously: to plan for them; to undertake training in communicating with the media for themselves and their immediate colleagues and subordinates; and to initiate good, positive, proactive relationships with journalists.

Conclusion

Good communication within health and social care does not just happen, it has to be planned for and managed. In times of rapid organizational change good communication – that is, reliable, timely and understandable communication – is an essential component of that change process.

Further reading

Adair J (1986) *Effective Team Building.* Gower, Aldershot.
Booth A (1988) *The Communications Audit. Guide for Managers.* Gower, Aldershot.
Ellis R and McLintock A (1994) *If You Take My Meaning.* Edward Arnold, London.
Evans D W (1986) *People, Communications & Organisations.* Pitman, London.
Fitzgerald N (1993) 'Time to break down the need-to-know barrier', *Scotsman*, March.
Industrial Society *Team Briefing Systems.* The Industrial Society, 3 Carlton Terrace, London SW17 5DG.

9

The manager meets the
customer/consumer

In this chapter we look at how and when we wish to involve patients and clients in planning and evaluating the service that is given; how to give a good level of customer care; who are our customers and clients.

Introduction

Nowadays the people that we work with are known as customers or consumers whether we work for British Rail (no longer a passenger) or the NHS (no longer a patient). Many people feel this is a derogatory way of looking at those that we care for, but there is an important lesson to be learnt from using this terminology. It helps us to focus on the fact that the people that are coming through the doors of a centre or clinic are not just users of our services, but human beings who have a right to an opinion and a say about what they are being subjected to.

In this context, we have to consider that there are internal and external customers for services. The internal customer is one who also works for the organization and could therefore be yourself when using a staff canteen or requesting help from the administration department. External customers are the people that we would recognize as patients, clients, residents and carers, i.e. those from outside our own organization. In considering getting feedback from customers, therefore, both groups have to be considered.

Why consult consumers?

One of the difficulties of providing care for others is that for the most part they do not choose to be in the situation where they need your help. Consider visitors to a museum or cinema – not only have they chosen to be there, but they may have paid to get in as well. It puts people in a very different type of relationship and makes them feel that they have more of a right to speak back to you.

The emphasis now in the service sector is on consulting with consumers. There have been charters which say this, management executives who say this, but most importantly it should be something that every care professional should *want* to do. Traditionally, professions have always known best and a lot of the resistance to consulting, particularly external consumers, is that many staff find it hard to come to terms with doing something differently because a 'lay person' tells them to.

This should not be what consulting consumers is about though. It is important for many reasons to consult consumers:

- to reaffirm patients and clients as the focus of the service;
- to inform purchasing and providing agendas;
- to involve people and encourage participation in decision making;
- to listen and hear what people have to say;
- to try to understand others' views and perceptions; and
- to gain knowledge from those who use the services.

There are probably many more good reasons, but these few show us what we have been missing for decades.

As with most ideas that will effect a sea change within the organization, consulting consumers will not work without the commitment to the process of all those involved. This means that you, as managers, have to be prepared to take part and take on board information that is gained through this process. In turn, your staff and your own managers all have to believe in the consultation.

But what if you are one of the consumers? How do you think that they will feel about this process? Why should they believe that we want to hear what they have to say after years of defensiveness and putting up barriers against perceived criticism? For years people have not even been asked what they think about our services, let alone whether they met their wants or needs. Now we have 'needs led services' (1990 NHS and Community Care Act) and purchasing or providing agendas. So all of a sudden there is supposed to be a well-informed and articulate public able to speak in language that planners and purchasers understand.

In many cases this might well be the case, but think of more disadvantaged sections of the population in terms of speaking up for themselves – people with learning difficulties or mental health problems. How can they be helped to take part in consultation?

Difficulties in consultation

One of the first points to make relates to the fact that everyone is wanting to ask questions of service customers these days, in order to assess standards and acceptability of service. This leads to fatigue or cynicism on behalf of those being consulted and also means that you need to be aware of other consultation initiatives within your organization.

Secondly, if you wish to consult your patients or clients, there can be difficulties with obtaining reliable and valid information. When you are using a service and something goes wrong, how easy do you find it to actually stand up and say something? How easy would you find it to make truthful comments if you were in the middle of receiving a course of counselling, support or treatment? As we have already mentioned, our customers in the caring professions are generally not receiving our service by choice. They come to us because they have some kind of difficulty which immediately puts them into a dependent role. People therefore have a fear of possible reprisal or feel that they may contribute to the disappearance of a service if they make critical or unfavourable remarks. Far easier then to try to say something non-committal or what you think the questioner wants to hear.

Ethical considerations must also be taken into account when consulting with others. If you wish to hold information in a database then you should be aware of the Data Protection Act and people's rights (see Chapter 13). You must also ensure that information you receive is treated with confidentiality and that anonymity is ensured if you are to get truthful answers.

Who sets the agenda?

Where do we start in terms of consultation? When a process is new to an organization it is not always easy to know where to start and decisions have to be made about one-off consultation or an on-going process through user panels or regular committees or discussion groups. Certain issues will need to be consulted on because the public themselves will be putting forward suggestions and complaints. It may be that an organizational customer satisfaction survey has been completed that tells us what things need attention. Local Health Councils and pressure groups all have their agendas and internally decisions have to be made about allocation of resources to services.

However, for many of us consultation will be at a much more local level – the patients and clients that you have everyday contact with (external customers) and referring agencies and colleagues (internal customers). Even if you just speak to them informally or monitor the comments that you are getting from people (in contrast to issuing questionnaires or carrying out interviews) you are tapping into your customers' expectations and attitudes about the service that you are providing. If we think of the customer as the person or agency to whom we provide a service, then it follows that we need to find ways of identifying their expectations and concerns about that service.

Many surveys have clearly shown up a degree of mismatch between the areas of the service which the professionals think do not 'come up to scratch' and the concerns expressed by patients or clients (*see* Case study 9.1)

Case study 9.1

> In an out-patients department in a hospital a short questionnaire was created for all patients coming through the clinics and they were asked to complete it whilst waiting for their appointment. The survey was undertaken for a complete week so that a variety of patients and clinics were covered.
>
> Staff thought that patients would comment unfavourably on waiting times, lack of time spent by staff with patients and lack of information about what was happening during the clinic. What they found, however, was that the three main areas of concern for patients were car parking difficulties, the decor of the waiting areas and poor sign-posting. Patients also reported very favourably on the friendliness and helpfulness of staff whom they saw clearly as 'overworked', but dealing with the situation to the best of their ability.

Two important issues come out of this short example. First that whilst patients did not find the same issues untenable, staff were able actually to address the items that were reported to be of importance once they knew what they were. Secondly, we need to be aware that as professionals we cannot always second guess what *is* of importance to patients/clients. This is of particular importance when trying to provide adequate information and a good standard of service. We need to know what our customers feel makes their contact with the service more acceptable as well as the areas that they do not understand and therefore need more explanation about.

What we must learn, and be prepared to accept and listen to is the creation of a 'shared agenda'. Professionals often feel unsure about consulting with customers as they feel threatened by the process and are convinced that their professional judgement is about to be questioned. In our experience, this is not the case, professional judgement is not routinely questioned, but rather, it is assumed. It is the mode and manner of delivery that is the focus of the shared attention.

How far can we meet customers' expectations?

So far we have been concentrating on the consultation process in order to assess others' views of our service. What now happens to the information that is collected and how does it affect the service that is delivered? Given that the desire to provide a quality service underpins most people's working practice, it is important at this stage to understand the nature of quality and the link between quality and standards.

In Chapter 12 there is a broader discussion of quality, but for now the problem that we shall concentrate on is that quality service is highly subjective. You only have to think of recommending a restaurant that *you* have enjoyed to someone else and the issue of shared values (or otherwise) is instantly illustrated. Thus, one way of dealing with these subjective variations is to seek to structure customers' expectations through a process of setting standards and this involves determining the level of service to be provided in an explicit, achievable and measurable way. By doing this, you are seeking to structure the expectation of the consumer, as well as making an explicit demand from your staff about what level of service is acceptable. Once achieved, as a manager you have set objectives and translated some of the subjectivity around service delivery into more tangible form.

Customer care

We have established that the whole point of consulting consumers is to improve the level of service that is provided. We have also discussed that one way of setting the shared agenda for this process between customers and professionals is to set standards that everyone can agree on – whether at a national level through patients charters etc. or at a local level through departmental standards. But how can you make sure that these theoretical promises are translated into action and therefore ensure that customers are cared for to a high standard?

The practice of providing customer care training is one way of addressing this issue. This has become increasingly important in recent years, although images of 'have a nice day' and 'sparkle classes' understandably have led some to view customer care with great cynicism, and it is important to work hard to dispel these gut reactions. In the public sector there is no difficulty in affirming that the 'customer' – whether patient, client or colleague – should be cared for. Indeed, this is the basic motivation for many professionals working in the public sector. The debate is about what customer care means in the public sector and the implications for our everyday practice.

What is customer care?

It is usually stated that customer care is about treating others as you would like to be treated yourself. This in itself, however, leaves the door open to a wide variety of behaviour and we have to work harder at customer care in order to ensure that people are treated as individuals and not just part of an organizational process. At one level customer care is about being friendly, helpful and courteous towards our customers, but on another level it is about communication of our underlying attitudes.

Activity

> Think of yourself in an everyday situation in which you are a customer, e.g. in a shop, restaurant or seeking the service of an electrician. Take five minutes to make a list of what you consider to be elements of a 'good' service and indicators of a 'poor' service.

In relation to a poor service, your list may include items such as:

- rudeness
- being ignored
- unkept promises, e.g. 'I'll come round at 3 pm'
- arrogance
- lack of information
- being patronized.

Your list of good indicators might include:

- helpfulness
- listening
- patience
- promptness
- courtesy
- being called by the right name.

The essential difference between these two lists can be summarized with reference to:

- appearance
- approach
- attitude.

Appearance

Positive impressions, particularly first impressions, make all the difference to our perception of a service. The person who answers the phone, the receptionist who greets us on arrival and the level/accuracy of signposting all provide an impression and instant feedback about the service that you are about to encounter. The use of name tags and a neat appearance, 'smart but appropriate', whether we like it or not, offer the superficial but significant first insight into the service. From our previous example, providing a pleasant waiting area with resasonably up-to-date magazines, for example, communicates that the organization cares enough to have dedicated some resource to this aspect of the service.

The problem with a lot of these examples is that if you work in a setting long enough, you learn to live with its shortcomings – you literally do not see them any more. Try to go into work one day as if it were for the first time and recapture your first impressions of the place. It is easy for people to argue that money spent on carpets could well have bought an extra computer but remember, to your customer, the carpets represent a significant contribution to their satisfaction with the service.

Approach

This aspect of customer care includes both behavioural and interpersonal issues. The way you behave towards another person clearly affects the way they behave toward you, i.e. behaviour breeds behaviour. If you greet a person in a positive, friendly and courteous manner then you increase the possibility that they will respond in a similar fashion. Equally if you are somewhat abrupt and fail to make eye contact, perhaps because you are busy and your mind is elsewhere, then the customer experiences this as lack of care and attention and will tend to respond in a similarly negative way. It costs nothing to smile and to acknowledge the presence of another person, regardless of how busy you are.

Attitude

Underpinning all of the issues relating to customer care are the attitudes held by members of staff and expressed through their appearance and approach. In situations where your customers are looking for some help, or seeking information, what we need to aim for is to find ways to say 'yes' rather than be tempted into saying why the request is not possible. There can be a tendency for busy members of staff to experience the demands of customers as an interruption to the task in hand. In one sense this is true, but this merely confirms that we should see people as pivotal to the service; they are, after all what the service is being provided for, rather than an unnecessary interruption to the smooth running of the organization.

When something goes wrong, e.g. a client is kept waiting for an appointment, it is all too easy to shrug your shoulders and blame someone else in the system rather than taking a collective responsibility for the experience of that individual and attempting to deal with the problem by giving an explanation and meeting their needs where possible. Remember that what people want above all is a solution to a problem, not further complications or abdication of responsibility.

Managing customer care

There are a number of things that you can do as a manager to try to develop good customer care in your team.

- Encourage all members of the team to view their service through the eyes of the customer.

- Help staff to evaluate aspects of the service in terms of approach, attitude and appearance.
- Identify with your team who are your internal and external customers.
- Discuss, agree and set standards of customer care in areas such as how you answer the telephone, waiting times, providing information, etc.
- Identify who in your team is particularly good at customer care and use them as an example for others.
- Be aware of and take responsibility for the overall level of customer care provided by your team, which includes providing support or coaching to improve standards for each individual where necessary.

Dealing with complaints

This is a particular aspect of customer care for which, in our experience, staff feel they need extra encouragement or support. It can be seen as the negative side of customer care, i.e. when the system has not met an individual's expectations. If good practice in customer care has been followed then this should minimize or reduce the number of complaints that your team will encounter – a good reason for improving everyone's customer care skills since this heads off the problem of complaints before they arise. A good example of this is to offer people explanations for a delay or problem before they feel they need to ask.

The basis of a complaint presented by a customer is that there is a mismatch between expectation and the service actually received. It is important, therefore, to let customers make their case. Do not cut them off when they approach with their complaint, and listen and respect the view of the customer even though you might think that it is misplaced. If necessary then take the step of apologizing on behalf of the organization. By doing this you have taken the first step in handling the complaint well.

Once you have heard what they have to say, the next step is to work with the customer to find a solution that is realistic and acceptable to you both. Quite often at this stage, courteous explanations are sufficient to satisfy a complainant and body language and calm non-verbal behaviour also reinforces the message that you are taking the complaint seriously. The issue here is moving from a defensive reaction when your service is challenged, to a proactive search for ways to solve the problems raised.

Despite all of this, you and your staff will encounter some customers who are plain aggressive or violent. This may be understandable because they are in a stressful situation or it may be because they are drunk or desperate. In this kind of situation, do not be afraid to seek help from one or more colleagues in order to diffuse the anger before the situation may be dealt with on a more even footing.

Finally, if the matter cannot be settled satisfactorily, it is important to bring to people's attention any organizational complaints procedures where they exist, so that they are made fully aware of their rights as a customer.

Conclusion

In this brief chapter we have tried to highlight some of the issues that surround the people who are central to our service, namely the external customers – that is, our patients and clients. Whether we wish to improve our knowledge of what constitutes an acceptable service through consultation with others, or try to improve their experience of what can be a traumatic event in their lives, the fact that the service is not delivered for ourselves has to be reinforced to everyone.

Further reading

McIver S (1991) *An Introduction to Obtaining the Views of Users of Health Services.* King's Fund Centre, London

National Health Service in Scotland and the Scottish Consumer Council (1994) *Consulting Consumers. A Guide to Good Practice.* HMSO, Scotland.

Shropshire Health Authority (1992) *Getting to the Core. A Practical Guide to Understanding Users' Experience in the Health Service.* Shropshire Health Authority in Conjunction with University of Birmingham.

Sykes W et al. (1992) *Listening to Local Voices. A Guide to Research Methods.* Nuffield Institute for Health Services Studies, Leeds and the Public Health Research and Resource Centre, Salford.

10

The manager as accountant

In this chapter we outline key areas of knowledge about costings that any manager in the health or social care services will need to have in terms of types of cost - direct and indirect, fixed and variable. We discuss apportionment and various ways of costing a treatment, together with an exercise.

Introduction

Someone once said that war is too important to be left to the generals. We might also say that accountancy is too important to be left to accountants. Accountancy is a highly complex subject and long study is required to master it. However those who aspire to manage effectively in health and social care need to have some degree of expertise in this field because of devolved budgets and financial planning. The aim of the next two chapters is to provide you with enough instruction in the matter of accountancy to manage effectively in the area of finance. Increasingly devolved management means that all managers will need to be familiar with these aspects of finance. It is not a subject that we can leave solely to others.

There are two broad divisions by which we might classify this area for our present purpose. These are costing and budgeting.

- *Costing* can be simply defined as the discovery of the actual costs of particular goods or services: for example, finding the cost of the removal of a kidney in a diabetic, or a 45 minute home visit by a district nurse to an elderly patient.
- *Budgeting*, which depends on costing, can equally simply be defined as the setting of standard or target costs for the future delivery of these same goods and services, after inefficiencies and incompetencies have been removed.

We have said that these are simple definitions, and as such, they are far from complete, but they are informative enough for our present purpose.

Costing

The rest of this chapter will be taken up with a demonstration of how to discover the cost of a particular good or service, in a specific setting. By specific setting we mean to draw attention to the fact that the cost of an identical procedure will be different if it is carried out in a nineteenth-century hospital in one city compared with an up-to-date hospital in another; and so also for all the other factors that influence cost in their great variety of specific settings.

This point is very relevant to the new ethos of competition that has been introduced into the health services in the UK: real difficulties occur when making such comparisons, as these often discriminate unfairly against individual hospitals and other services. You only have to look at the production of league tables to realize the difficulties that abound and the outcry that is raised when direct comparisons are made from one setting to another.

Until recently, costing individual treatments was not done in the health and social services, and only now is a national costing project trying to ensure uniformity of approach. Certainly, there is no dispute about the necessity of costing. In order to understand the situation clearly we might look briefly at the reasons for costing, which we present below as the 'three Cs':

- *Control:* Only by knowing the costs of each area of health care, and of each type of treatment can limited resources be properly managed.

- *Comparison:* Finding out what the costs of the same episodes of care are enable us to compare different centres, so that inefficiencies might be exposed and corrected.

- *Charging:* In private health care and under the new regime in the NHS and social work where there are 'purchasers' and 'providers', it is necessary to 'charge' for episodes of care that constitute service provision. Even where the costs are paid under a block contract, it is necessary to know what these costs are, so that the proper charge can be negotiated. The charge is not paid by the patient, although some social care clients pay for services such as meals on wheels or day care, but in either case charges are paid in respect of the patient/client, so it will be helpful in all the discussion that follows, if it is borne in mind that eventually all the costs of a service, even the cost of drainage, interest charges, legal fees, malpractice penalties, must be charged some way or another against all individuals who use the service, whoever actually pays.

Types of cost

Direct and indirect costs

The first distinction to be made is that costs can be *direct* or *indirect*. The difference is important, and easily explained. Direct costs are those that belong exclusively to the unit, or department, or 'cost centre' that is being studied; if we are concerned, say, with an acute admission ward in a large psychiatric hospital, then the salary of the nurses who work exclusively in that department would be a direct cost, but the salary of the chief executive of the hospital as a whole would be an indirect cost. The importance of this distinction, as we shall see, lies in the need to find a way of sharing ('apportioning') the cost of the chief executive's salary fairly amongst all the departments of the hospital. No such problem arises with the nurses' salaries, because they are borne in their totality by the department, in that they are exclusive to the department, and shared by no other; that is, they are 'direct'.

Activity

> With that bare definition, arrange the following mixed list into *direct* and *indirect* costs in relation to an acute admission department:
>
> psychiatrists' salaries; depreciation on payroll computers; cost of stationery for administration; local authority rates; chief executive's salary; cost of drugs; salaries of department nurses; depreciation on ward equipment; salaries of the general administrative staff; cost of beds and chairs; upkeep of grounds.

Your lists should look like this:

Direct	*Indirect*
psychiatrists' salaries	depreciation on payroll computers
cost of drugs	cost of stationery for administration
salaries of department nurses	local authority rates
deprecation on ward equipment	chief executive's salary
cost of beds and chairs	salaries of general administration staff
	upkeep of grounds

(... and many other direct and indirect costs).

Although in most cases the distinction is clear, there may be some difficulties here and there in deciding whether a cost is direct or indirect. Take, for example, the cost of cleaning in a general hospital. In most hospitals cleaning is carried out on a general basis by a central unit, serving the entire hospital; clearly this is an indirect cost to the various departments. But it may be that in the theatre and the intensive care unit the cleaning is carried out by a small specialist team who concentrate on these areas alone, and do not work for any other department. In this case the costs are direct, and have to be borne in their entirety by the department – there is no question of sharing these costs with any other.

Fixed and variable costs

The next important distinction to make is between items called fixed and variable costs.

Fixed costs

These are costs that remain unaltered, even although the number of patients/clients rises or falls. If local authority business rates are £10 000 in one year for a local social work department, and if the number of clients increases by 5 per cent the next year, the rates will not be increased for this reason, nor will they be reduced if the number of clients falls. The rates are fixed. Of course the rates may change for other reasons – inflation, for example – but they will not vary because of and in proportion to a change in client numbers. Similarly, interest chargeable on money spent for medical equipment will be fixed despite changes in patient numbers, as will a number of other costs such as money spent on training. A consultant's salary will be fixed, in that he or she will expect to be paid the same, even if patient numbers decline, and, conversely, the hospital will expect the consultant to work for the previously agreed salary even if numbers rise (the advent of performance-related pay may change this to a certain extent, but this merely goes to illustrate the principle).

Variable costs

Variable costs vary in direct proportion to the number of patients/clients, that is to volume of activity. They represent costs incurred in respect to physical things such as drugs and dressings and so on, that are directly used or absorbed by individual patients. If the number of patients rises by 5 per cent, it is likely that the use of drugs will rise by 5 per cent. If the number of patients drops by 3 per cent, it is likely that the use of diagnostic tests will drop by 3 per cent. The fact that variable costs can be connected with individual patients/clients makes them easily measured. The cost of, say, a dose of insulin is fairly easy to determine; it is basically the price paid to the pharmaceutical company; the number of doses a patient gets in a given period of time is exactly known – it must be recorded for clinical reasons. Therefore the charge with respect to that patient for insulin can be exactly and readily determined.

There is, however, a slight problem with regard to variable costs which are relatively small. This refers to things that are given to, used for, or applied to patients/clients, that may not be recorded individually, e.g. thermometers; these are small inexpensive items that may be used a large number of times on several patients before they are lost or broken. In this case such costs, since they cannot be readily attributed to patients individually, and also since they apply to most patients more or less equally, can be lumped together, and the average cost per patient-day computed.

Take this example. Say the total cost of these 'sundry supplies' in a year amounted to £125 000; there are 50 000 patient-days, then the cost of these per patient-day is £2.50 – a relatively small amount. (This is a form of apportionment, which will be described later in connection with indirect costs.)

Semi-fixed and semi-variable costs

Having now described both fixed and variable costs, we can observe that not all costs fall into one or the other category; there are such things as semi-fixed, or semi-variable costs, which as the name suggests share the characteristics of both categories.

A familiar example is the telephone bill. If in a quarter you receive a phone bill amounting to, say, £170; on examining it you will find that £9 of this is a fixed (standing) charge; the rest is variable, depending on the number of units used at a certain rate per unit. So, even if you doubled your phone usage, the fixed charge would stay the same, and only the element representing the variable charge would double; if you did not use the phone at all in the next quarter, you would still have to pay the £9 standing charge.

Another point to be noted in relation to fixed costs is this: while they do not vary with activity, this situation holds good only over a certain range of activity. A social worker may see 400 clients a year; if the number increases to 420, his or her pay is likely to remain the same; the same holds true for a decline in the number. But if the number of clients presenting increases substantially, there comes a point where the social worker just cannot cope; another (possibly part time) social worker would have to be appointed or (to be more realistic) the prospective new patients will be relegated to a waiting list. In other words, the fixed cost of that one social worker's salary suddenly becomes unfixed, and increases to a higher level. However, this higher level now becomes a fixed cost in relation to the range of the number of patients the new 'social worker capacity' can support.

As semi-fixed or semi-variable costs introduce quite large complications into our calculations of charges they will be ignored from here on, so that we can clearly expound the principles of costing in this chapter. Further advice can be taken and these complications can readily be included in real situations if need be.

Apportionment

Now we come to the problem of sharing the indirect costs between the various departments of a hospital or social work centre. It will help in understanding this to repeat the point made earlier – that all costs, direct or indirect, must be attributed in the end to the individual patients / clients and their episodes of care. With this in mind then, how can we tell how much the patients say in a medical department, whether it is respite care, pneumonia or unstable diabetes, have to be charged as their share of the chief executive's salary, rates, insurance, and all the other indirect costs?

Apportionment is one of the main problems in costing, it is the term used to describe how these indirect costs should be shared. There are two main routes to calculating apportionment.

Option 1

This is a traditional method by which a means of measuring the absorption of a particular service would be chosen, and the costs would be apportioned on that basis. A good example is heating, as shown in Case study 10.1

Case study 10.1

> If the heating is all done by a central plant then the annual cost of heating an entire hospital complex could be easily determined, and from that point the cost per cubic metre per year could be easily calculated. From there, knowing the volume of the department in question, that department's share of the total could be simply determined. If the total cost is, say, £1 000 000, and the volume of the hospital is 500 000 cubic metres, then the cost per cubic metre per year is obviously £2. If the volume of the medical department is 60 000 cubic metres, then the annual cost to be apportioned to that department would be 60 000 × £2 = £120 000.

The same principle could be used for other facilities, such as cleaning, upkeep of grounds, administrative services, and so on; but obviously, a different unit would have to be used, for example, area not volume for cleaning, staff numbers for payroll administration, and whatever is appropriate for others. These when added together indicate the total indirect cost that the department in question must pay towards all the general costs of the hospital.

Drawbacks to this method

As we have said, this is the traditional method and it is fairly straightforward (even if painstaking). However useful it might have been in the past though, it has its drawbacks. These do not need to be discussed here, except to mention the most important factor, which is that there is a further need to apportion these costs on from the department to the patient. This is in observance of the fundamental principle we have already established that 'the patient pays'. What base might we use to take this large departmental indirect cost and share it out fairly amongst all the patients it treats? Patients require a wide range of treatments, and it would not seem appropriate to charge them all the same flat amount for indirect costs.

If a department treats 5000 patients in a year it would be simple to charge each of them one five-thousandth of the total, but that would be far from an exact or 'fair' measure of the amount of the various services the individual patients 'use'.

Option 2

It would, of course, be impossible to measure exactly, but an acceptably accurate, and yet simple method would be to use the concept of time – that is to charge patients/clients according to the time they spend in the department or unit in question.

If it is a ward, then a patient-day could be the unit of charge, and if it is an operating theatre, then it could be patient-hour. So then, in the simple example regarding heating already quoted, if the total number of patient - days in that year were 250 000, then dividing the £1 000 000 cost by this number would give £4 per patient-day; for a length of stay of 4 days the charge to that patient for heating would be £16, and for a patient in hospital for 10 days, £40. Of course, instead of recording a separate charge for each of the many indirect services, the total of all of them would be established, and that figure used to produce a charge per patient-day for all indirect costs.

Using the concept of time to settle on an appropriate charge will avoid the wearisome task of calculating areas, volumes, or whatever other measurement is appropriate, and also avoid the two-stage process of calculating the departmental charge, then the share of that to be borne by the individual case. Instead we can proceed immediately from the total cost of general services and facilities to the charge for any particular patient.

Costing an episode of care

We now have to consider the application of the above points and principles. As we are trying to grasp the basics of costing, we shall use a surgical procedure as an example, since this is a discrete episode of care which can be identified. Let us consider, therefore, the calculation of the cost of having your appendix removed (appendicectomy). This is a standard procedure, and we shall treat it as such in this costing process, but it must be remembered that there could be non-standard situations, such as if the patient were also a diabetic, which could change the cost picture as the patient's stay would involve more complex treatment or their time in hospital could be extended.

In the following example the concepts of interest and depreciation are introduced, which until recently were ignored in the consideration of health and social care costs. For the moment accept these, and we shall discuss them later as 'capital charging'.

Now we are in a position to carry through an actual costing exercise. Note that the values used in this are not necessarily taken from a real situation, but they are realistic. As stated we shall use an appendicectomy as the vehicle of the demonstration. The patient in question will be admitted to a general ward for one day. The next day he or she will be prepared for the operation, undergo the operation, spend a few hours in the recovery room, then be taken back to the ward, where he or she will remain for that day, and three more – a total of five days in the ward.

The calculations are shown below, followed by a series of points which discuss various issues pertaining to the exercise.

A. Direct fixed costs:
Annual time spent on operations by the surgical team: 1250 hours

			Total	Running total
Annual payroll of the unit			£490 000	£490 000
Capital costs of unit	Depreciation	£50 000		
	Interest	£30 000	£80 000	
Other direct fixed costs		£30 000	£30 000	
Total direct fixed costs				£600 000

1250 hours of clinical activity incur a cost of
£600 000;
therefore 1 hour costs 600 000/1250 = £480
An uncomplicated appendicectomy takes

1 hour so an appendicectomy costs 480 × 1 =	£480	£480
B. Variable costs	£120	£600

Fluids, anaesthetic materials, disposable instruments, etc.

C. Ward charge:
Calculated on same principle as A and B:
£85 per patient-day, so ward charge for
this patient:

85 × 5 =	£425	£1 025

D. Indirect fixed costs:

Total general costs for hospital	£10 500 000		
Total patient-days	150 000		

so, cost per patient-day:
10 500 000/150 000 = £70

and charge to this patient 70 × 5 days =	£350	£1 375
Total cost of uncomplicated appendicectomy		£1 375

This system can be used for any kind of health care treatment, as it is in principle used for any product or service. Another example will be given later, as well as an exercise, which will help to consolidate the technique in your mind. However as mentioned, a number of points have to be made in relation to this:

1. The above calculation depends on past activity; it shows what the cost *has been* and not what the cost *should be* in the future. This is a matter to be treated under budgeting.
2. The cost calculated above is not necessarily what the charge should be; that is, no allowance appears to have been made for surplus (or profit, as it would be called in the commercial sector).
3. As will be further discussed under budgeting, the computed charge may not in fact be chargeable – that is competing institutions may charge less, thus inhibiting you from applying the charge you wish. This problem will be discussed under marginal costing and pricing, which will come under budgeting.
4. The amount of the charge in respect of indirect fixed costs is especially difficult, since it depends on the total patient-days 'produced' by the hospital. If these had been less than the 150 000 in the example, the charge would be higher; if they were more the charge would be less. This, again, is a problem faced by all organizations – predicting the volume of production.
5. A crucial element is the 1250 hours of clinical activity used in the calculation. A moment's thought will reveal that this is far from being the total time employed for a surgeon or any other full-time member . This is more likely to be in the region of 37.5 hours a week, or, to allow for possible overtime, 40 hours a week. Multiply this by 46 working weeks in the year, and we get 1840. Why the difference? Because some of the working week is spent not on actual direct contact with the patient in the theatre or operating room, but on other activities, such as writing up records, attending meetings, research, consulting with each other and even coffee breaks. But this time is paid for, and must therefore be charged to the patient.

    So, in taking the total cost inclusive of these non-clinical functions, and dividing it by the clinical time we get a figure (£480 an hour) which will effectively ensure that the entire cost is met by charging the patients according to the measurable time spent on them. If we simply calculate the hourly rate of pay, and apply only that to the clinical time how will the money paid for the report writing, coffee breaks, etc. be produced? (dividing the £600 000 by the employed time, 1840 hours, gives only £326 an hour).
6. Payroll, of course, includes not only the salary of the employee, but the associated superannuation and National Insurance costs incurred by the institution.

7. Capital charging (depreciation and interest) will be dealt with under budgeting.

As suggested before, this system may be used for any commercial or social activity where money costs are involved, and in any branch of that activity. Even in the wide range of health care activity there is no situation to which it cannot be applied. To illustrate this, and to give you a chance to apply what you have learned, the following exercise is offered.

Activity

An occupational therapy department is situated in a large general hospital, and occupies 1.2 per cent of the area. This is the proportion of indirect costs of the hospital that is to be charged to the department.

The department is supervised by a senior occupational therapist whose salary is £22 000 a year. She is also in charge of another OT unit in a health centre to which she applies 20 per cent of her time.

There are four other OTs in the department whose pay averages £18 500 a year, three OT helpers with an average pay of £8900, and a clerical assistant/receptionist, whose pay is £7800 a year.

Employer's National Insurance and superannuation contributions amounting to 14 per cent must be added to the salaries.

An 84-year-old woman in-patient with severe osteoarthritis is due to be discharged, and a home assessment is to be made for her. This will involve a total of 60 minutes of direct patient time, and a further 90 minutes of patient-related time, including travel. A jug-kettle tipper costing £8.50, and a pair of tap turners costing £3.50 will have to be supplied to her. Travel amounts to an average of 6 miles per assessment, using the OT's own car, for which she receives £0.33 per mile.

Sundry supplies are used by the department at an annual cost of £14 400.

The hospital has general overheads amounting to £10 363 500, including capital charges. The annual number of patient-hours, both direct and patient-related hours, that the department provides is 6345.

Calculate the cost of this assessment.

Note. This exercise includes a few ideas that have not been directly discussed in the text, for example, what do you do with the fact that the supervisor spends 20 per cent of her time in another unit? However, you are now familiar with the principles of costing, and you should be able to decide how to resolve these problems.

Solution

Total patient-hours 6345

This patient 60 + 90 minutes = 150 minutes = 2.5 hours

Direct fixed costs:

Pay: Supervisor: 80% of 22 000 =	£17 600	
OT's 4 × 18 500 =	£74 000	
Assistants 3 × 8900 =	£26 700	
Clerk	£7 800	
Total pay	£126 100	
Add 14% for NI and superannuation	£17 654	
	£143 754	

Cost per hour 143 754/6345 = £22.66

Cost for this patient £22.66 × 2.5 hours =   £56.65

Variable costs:

Sundries: 14 400/6345 = 2.27 per hour × 2.5 hours =	£5.67
Travel: 6 miles x £0.33 =	£1.98
Materials: £8.50 + 3.50 =	£12.00

Indirect fixed costs:

Overheads: £10 363 500 × 1.2% = £124 362

Overhead cost per hour = 124 362/6345 = £19.60

and for this patient £19.60 × 2.5 hours =   £49.00

Total charge: £125.30

You might have tackled this problem according to a different layout from the above. That does not matter as long as you have the same answer, allowing, perhaps, for small differences due to rounding.

Further reading

Department of Health (1987) *Health Service Costing Returns.* London.
NHS in Scotland (1994-5) *Scottish Health Service Costs.* Edinburgh.

11

The manager as budget holder

In this chapter we examine various ways of drawing up a budget, establishing the 'target'; distinguishing between capital and recurrent costs together with an examination of ward budgeting with various examples and an exercise.

So far we have looked at the principles of costing, and the method of determining the cost of a particular form of treatment. For this purpose we took an appendicectomy as an example, and worked through the costing process. It is important to remember that this procedure was based on data derived from past experience, e.g. the number of clinical hours actually worked in the past year, the actual payroll of the surgical team in the past year, and so on.

Definition

Budgeting, in a sense, is the opposite of that. In budgeting we are concerned with a situation that has not happened yet – with next year. It might be said that 'well next year should be like last year, so there should be little difference'. This, however, would be contrary to the principle of budgeting, because since we are concerned with the future, our natural human inclination is to improve on things. Indeed, it is not merely an inclination, but a necessity to continuously strive to improve things in whatever field, but particularly in health and social services today (*see* Chapter 12 on quality management). So we may define budgeting simply as planning to achieve a given target. This is vague, but still, it is a useful definition to bear in mind because it highlights two fundamental things about budgeting, namely it is about a target and it is about a plan.

Traditional budgeting

Two further points should be made at this stage. The first is that until recently budgeting in health and social services was largely conducted in the manner we rejected a few sentences ago. That is to say, budgets for one year were simply an extension of previous years' activities, with no real attempt to set a target of performance, or devise a plan to reach it (nor indeed in many cases was there any real attempt even to assess or evaluate last year's performance). The attitude was simply that we got through last year pretty well, so if we do the same next year that should be adequate. Well, this approach probably would be adequate if all notion of advance and improvement were abandoned. But nowadays we are not, and cannot afford to be so casual and unimaginative – where an activity or facility is new a special problem arises in particular, since there has been no previous experience to guide us.

The second point to be made is that for many people in health and social services, budgeting also meant being allocated a sum of money (the 'budget'), and having to ensure that they did not over or underspend it. This narrow accounting function did nothing to encourage independent thought and enterprise, and a search for efficiency. As will be seen, a central feature of budgeting is that the budget holder should be involved in formulating the target and the plan, not just be told from on high how much is available and to get on with it – the 'Zeus' approach to management (*see* Chapter 2).

Past performance as a guide

Although we have suggested that a budget should not merely be a carbon copy of previous years' activities, but should be an improvement, this does not mean that past performance is irrelevant. Actually, the only way we know what we are capable of is to know what we have achieved in the past. So discovering past costs, which we investigated in the last chapter, is vitally important, even if only to decide they were excessive and should be reduced. Reductions made in this way are known as 'efficiency savings', and nowadays are actually expected each year by increasing numbers of health and social care authorities.

The budgeting process

The first step is to decide on the volume of activity to be achieved. This simplistic, and rather crude way of putting it disguises the fact that caring 'activity' involves treating *real* people suffering from a *real* disease or disability. But it is a useful and succinct way of expressing what is really large numbers of people with many different conditions, each requiring a particular application of skill, knowledge and facilities. For this reason it is necessary to start off the budgeting process at the very beginning of the scale, namely with the smallest unit that can be managed as an individual entity. In other words, we cannot budget for an entire hospital without first budgeting for all its smallest parts, and then gathering these individual budgets together and integrating them (then possibly modifying them, if they cannot all be met in their entirety).

Money as a way of measuring value

Although we tend to think of budgeting as a financial process, it is important to remember that money is only a way of measuring value. When we speak of a budget as amounting to so much money we are really speaking of the things that can be done with that money – the numbers of nurses or social workers that can be employed, the type of facilities, the quantity of various drugs and medicines, and so on. This becomes all the more apparent, and unavoidable when we start to draw up a budget.

We must start with a target, which would usually be the number of clients we aim to serve, and the standard of their care; numbers and quality must be considered together. Of course, while numbers can be readily understood by a lay person or an accountant, the idea of quality of care is more subtle, and can really only be decided by people experienced in providing that care. This is what was meant earlier when we mentioned that the person responsible for running the unit (that is, implementing the budget) should be involved in constructing the budget in the first place. So, since neither the writer nor (probably) you, the reader, is in a position to define quality in relation to all possible care, we must be content to leave that to the actual devisors of the budget, and merely point out its fundamental importance.

Mechanics of drawing up a budget

Now to start on the actual mechanics of drawing up a budget. Since we have already used the idea of an appendicectomy in our study of costing, it will be appropriate to carry over the same idea to illustrate the budgeting process.

Below is a simple representation of a budget, followed by an explanation of the various steps. We have numbered these steps for clarity.

Budget for surgical unit
1. Target in clinical hours, annually: 1290

2. Direct fixed costs			
(a) Payroll			£300 000
(b) Capital	i. Depreciation	£50 000	
	ii. Interest	£40 000	£90 000
(c) Other			£55 000
3. Variable costs			£37 000
Total			£482 000

1. Establish the target

This would initially be expressed in terms of the different kinds of operation that the unit in question would undertake. The numbers of these various cases that are likely to be presented in the financial year in question should be established. The probable time taken for each of these has to be determined, with, crucially, due consideration for the desired quality of the work. At this stage some kind of allowance must also be made for more difficult cases.

Further, in considering the time allocated this must include not only the time the patient is in surgery, but also the time taken on the part of the team in preparation, and afterwards in whatever post-operative tasks must be undertaken, before a start can be made on the next patient. In the end we will have a list of the various cases, their numbers, and the average time allowed for each. Add all of the times together and we will have a number of hours, say, 1500, which represents the 'clinical time' that the envisaged patients will require.

We must also recognize, as has been intimated already, that time must be allowed for non-clinical functions, such as report writing, record-making, training, going to conferences, time off for illness and even coffee breaks (which contribute to the quality of the work), and this time must be added.

Suppose, in the judgement of the budgetsetters, all of these various requirements can be efficiently met in one-third of the time allocated for operations, that is, in this example, 500 hours. This means that the team will individually need to work 2000 hours a year. But the standard working year is only some 1725 hours. So, unless overtime is introduced, which will raise hourly costs, and possibly impair quality, the target will have to be modified, and a new and smaller mix of operations contemplated, which will efficiently fill the time available; or possibly some of the non-clinical activities might be cut back, but this too could affect quality.

A surgeon would no doubt find a number of other considerations that should be included in the above; but since this brief account of budgeting is intended for general use, and since each reader will want to apply it to his or her own situation – physiotherapy, radiography, health visiting, community care work – and will supply his or her own expertise, then this simple outline should be sufficient. Let us say that, in the end, it is decided that the team will be capable of supplying 1290 clinical hours at the required level of quality, and a further third for non-clinical work, giving a total of 1720. The target has now been set at 1290 clinical hours, representing a certain mix of operations.

There could be other restrictive situations (known as limiting factors), such as lack of facilities, or even lack of clients, but for the present example the limiting factor of staff has been used.

2. Direct fixed costs

(a) Payroll

In so far as we have already established the clinical hours, we will also have considered the numbers of the various personnel required for this service. Again, the exact make-up is a matter for the professionals in charge of the budget, and they will consider what disciplines, and what number and grade of these disciplines will be needed on the team, i.e. the skill mix. Let us say that it is decided that for the proper level of expertise, quality of service, and cost effectiveness there will be required a specialist, a senior registrar, a consultant anaesthetist, a junior anaesthetist, a scrub nurse, and two theatre nurses.

From this point, knowing their annual salaries, and adding the employer's pension contribution, and National Insurance contribution (about 8 per cent and 10 per cent respectively), their total cost can be readily calculated.

(b) Capital

This is a rather controversial subject because it has been largely ignored in health and social services until the reforms of the early 1990s, but then costing in general has been a somewhat arcane subject. Let us say a few words about the meaning of capital and also bear in mind that the word has two different meanings. The first, which is probably the meaning most people think of, is the total money value of the investment necessary to build and equip the hospital (or clinic, unit, factory, road, bridge – whatever the facility is that we are concerned with). In the second meaning, capital represents the actual physical things themselves. In this study we shall usually be speaking of the money value, but always be ready to ascertain which meaning is intended.

Distinguishing capital and recurrent costs   At this point it will be useful to distinguish more exactly between capital (that is, long-term) costs and recurrent (daily) costs. A motor car is a useful model to use. The capital costs of a car will be the initial buying price, and any major costs such as providing a new set of tyres after two or three years. The recurrent costs will be petrol, oil, normal maintenance, insurance and road tax.

A rule of thumb is that if the thing bought will last more than one year it is a capital item; if, on the other hand, it will be used up within a year it will be recurrent.

This is a rule of convenience, and obviously there could be indeterminate cases; for example, should the air filter in a car be treated as a recurrent cost or a capital cost? This would usually last more than a year, and would therefore be a capital item, but since it is such a relatively small cost, then it is more convenient just to treat it as recurrent, and save the trouble of calculating and recording annual depreciation (discussed below).

Activity

Classify the following costs as recurrent or capital:

social workers' salaries; lighting; crockery in cafeteria; new heating equipment; minibus for community centre; nurses' uniforms; TV and video for crèche; employer's pension contributions; local authority rates; purchase of site for nursing home; photo-copying machine; supply of assessment forms; liability insurance.

Your lists should look like this:

Capital	*Recurrent*
new heating equipment	social workers' salaries
minibus for community centre	lighting
TV and video for crèche	crockery in cafeteria
purchase of site for nursing home	nurses' uniforms
photo-copying machine	employer's pension contributions
	local authority rates
	supply of assessment forms
	liability insurance

There are two broad costs of capital: *depreciation* and *interest*.

Depreciation   This is the easiest of the two concepts to consider. It simply means the wear and tear on the physical parts of the facility. To take a simple example, if you build a new health centre at a cost of, say, £200 000 that money has to be repaid through the operation of the centre, that is by the patients/clients somehow. Now how should this cost be apportioned amongst the various patients? By dividing it on a patient-day basis over the patients in the first year of the centre's operation? Plainly this would be unfair, unreasonable and impossible. The capital cost should be divided 'fairly' over all the patients treated during the total life of the centre. In other words, we should calculate the annual cost of the centre, then apportion this on a patient-day basis year by year.

We have already spent a good deal of time talking about indirect fixed costs; well, the amount of wear and tear incurred by the centre each year is just another indirect fixed cost. How do we calculate this? There are a few ways, but the best for our purpose is simply to divide the total capital cost by the length of time the health centre will last; if it is reckoned that the buildings and facilities will last, say, 60 years, then the supposed £200 000 total cost previously mentioned, when divided by 60, will give an annual cost of £3333. This, then, may be taken as the amount to be added to the other indirect fixed costs for the year in question. The word *depreciation* is used to denote this sum. This, in other words, is a kind of *apportionment* applied over the number of years, which is then further apportioned over the number of patient-days within that year.

Needless to say the length of life of a health centre cannot be known until it is actually demolished; so, because we have to apportion its cost on an annual basis right from its first year, we have to estimate this as well as we can; further, some parts of a health centre have a different life span from others. The buildings are likely to last longer than the standby generators, or the boiler equipment; and these will last longer than the computers, so it follows that the depreciation of all of these different facilities has to be calculated separately, then added together to give the total annual depreciation – a tedious job, but not intellectually difficult.

For different departments within the centre the equipment of various kinds, used exclusively for that unit will also have to be calculated and the depreciation determined (that is, the direct capital cost). Let us say that for the present example, the total cost of the equipment and any other exclusive capital items is £20 000, and the estimated life is 10 years; this gives a figure of £2000 for depreciation for the budget calculation in question.

Interest   The more difficult concept in relation to capital is that of interest. Why should this capitalist idea be applied to a public, or 'free' system of care? Well, let us imagine for a start that we are speaking only of a commercial care operation, of which there are many in various parts of the world, and in the UK. The money for this service must be provided from somewhere. If it comes from a bank, then that bank will charge interest, and this interest must inevitably be regarded as an indirect fixed cost, not essentially different from depreciation, administration salaries, and all the rest. It follows that if a private enterprise, instead of borrowing, provides the funds from its own resources to set up the operation, it would do this only in order to receive a reward in the shape of profit (also a kind of 'interest') for doing so. In other words, the funds would not be forthcoming, and the facility would never be provided, unless a certain level of profit were in prospect. This level of profit is known as the return on capital.

If we now accept that private care establishments must charge an amount that represents the required return to their funders (among their various other costs), then it follows that even public institutions must do the same. Why so? Because not-for-profit institutions may also have to borrow money and therefore pay interest. Even when the money, or some of it, is provided by charity or the state, they must take into account the interest that the charity or the state must pay for borrowing the money, or the amount they forgo in not banking or otherwise investing it.

To wind up this argument without it getting too complicated, let us say that interest is a cost of capital like depreciation, which must be charged to the hospital, or facility and eventually to the client, in order to pay for the cost of providing the money which in turn provides the facilities.

What is the rate of interest, or the rate of return, that should be charged? This too is a problem, and is influenced by the inflation rate, but the British

Treasury figure has varied between 5 per cent and 8 per cent a year: the latter seems a more realistic figure, and will be used in these discussions.

In the analysis above, we have assumed a capital cost of just under £500 000 for the direct capital of the surgical unit; 8 per cent of this as interest provides a direct fixed cost, i.e. £40 000 for the year.

The fact that the lives of items of physical capital have to be estimated introduces a certain imprecision in costing and budgeting. Inflation also would tend to distort the picture. But these are complications that can be reduced by cautious judgement, even if they cannot be eradicated altogether. In sum, the matter of capital charging is a serious problem, but not such as to detain us too long in this general study of budgeting.

(c) Other

The items included under this heading, although they might amount to a considerable sum, represent a number of smaller costs, such as maintenance of equipment, consultation, postage, travel, which are exclusive to this unit and not general to the hospital (that is, they are direct).

3. Variable costs

These have already been explained in the last chapter. They are costs that vary directly with the clients, and refer to the actual costs of drugs administered to the patient, or appliances supplied to the client – all costs that can be individually identified. Included here also would be the cost of small, usual items which would be tedious to record, and which consequently it would be reasonable to apportion equally to each client on a patient-day basis, or by some other appropriate measure.

Budgetary control

However carefully a budget might be constructed there is always the possibility that it might not be followed exactly, and even that it might go awry. It is not unusual for the money allocated for a particular budget to peter out before the end of the financial year with the consequent embarrassing, annoying and even distressing postponements and cancellations.

Proper budgetary control should avoid this. Budgetary control implies two things. First, continuous *monitoring* of the budget, and second, *variance analysis.*

Monitoring

Basically, this means a frequent, regular check on the budget throughout the year to ensure that it is not beginning to deviate from the plan. For this reason it is necessary to take the annual budget, and divide it into regular periods of time – typically, monthly periods.

The simple way to do this is dividing by twelve; if, soon after the month in question ends, a comparison is made between what was budgeted for that month, and what was actually spent, we can know whether we are on target or not. If we are not, the cause can be investigated, and the situation corrected. We have referred to this as the simple way, but it is really too simple for a sophisticated budgeter, although it is a quick and useful way of explaining the system. The better way, and more in keeping with scientific budgeting, is to recognize the obvious fact that activity and expenditure in any organization varies in intensity from month to month, and even day to day. So, using the data already collected to construct the underlying annual budget, a series of monthly budgets should be drawn up, showing the anticipated activity, and the consequent costs. It will be convenient, even if slightly uneven, to use calendar and not 4-week months for this purpose. The fact that we are going to draw these up on the basis of actual activity and expenditure, and not on the basis of arithmetical twelfths, makes this all the more justifiable. Let us use two theoretical budgets for a ward – one representing the annual budget and the other a monthly budget of June as a model. They might look like this:

Annual budget for an acute medical ward:
1. Average daily number of patients: 27
2. (a) Annual payroll for nursing staff £450 000
   (b) Annual payroll for other staff £137 000
3. Annual cost of supplies £79 000
4. Capital charges:
   (a) depreciation £30 000
   (b) interest .... £24 000 .... £54 000
Total direct costs £720 000

Budget for June (30 days):
1. Average daily number of patients: 25
2. (a) Monthly payroll for nursing staff £34 245
   (b) Monthly payroll for other staff £10 425
3. Monthly cost of supplies £6 015
4. Capital charges £4 110
Total direct costs £54 795

Since the monthly budgets are, naturally, based on activity, then the number of patients is fundamental. Notice that in this case the average daily number of patients for this month is only 25, reflecting anticipated seasonal variations. Also, June having 30 days gives us a total number of patient-days of 750 (25 × 30).

The financial values of this monthly budget are calculated simply by applying the cost per patient-day already implicit in the annual budget. To do this we note that the annual patient-days are targeted to be 27 × 365; which gives us 9855. Dividing the individual annual amounts by this number gives us the following figures:

			Cost per patient-day
1.	Average daily number of patients: 27		
2.	(a) Annual payroll for nursing staff	£450 000	£45.66
	(b) Annual payroll for other staff	£137 000	£13.90
3.	Annual cost of supplies	£79 000	£8.02
4.	Capital charges:		
	(a) depreciation £30 000		
	(b) interest £24 000	£54 000	£5.48
Total direct costs		£720 000	£73.06

Now, apply these daily costs to the budget for June, taking into account the smaller average number of patients (which gives 750 patient-days), thus:

1.	Average daily number of patients: 25		
2.	(a) Monthly payroll for nursing staff	(45.66 × 750) =	£34 245
	(b) Monthly payroll for other staff	(13.90 × 750) =	£10 425
3.	Monthly cost of supplies	(8.02 × 750) =	£6 015
4.	Capital charges	(5.48 × 750) =	£4 110
Total direct costs			£54 795

Variance analysis

After all this work where are we? Simply in the position of being able to compare our budget with the actual results when we have completed our work for June, and have gathered the data. Suppose (as is not unlikely) that the actual results – the 'out-turn' – are different from the budget. Suppose the total out-turn is £60 643. We can immediately say: 'Something's gone wrong. We've overspent by nearly £6000. Thank goodness we've discovered this now, and not next February when the overspend might amount to £60 000 or more.'

But what has gone wrong? We cannot tell right away, but we can set about a variance analysis exercise to pinpoint the area or areas of overspend, i.e. look at how the actual budget compares with the projected budget. What we have to do here is break down the £60 643 into the actual expenditure on the individual items and compare these with their budgeted amounts. This comparison, then, might look like this:

Variance analysis for June:

		Budget	Out-turn	Variance
1.	Average daily number of patients	25	26	1A
2.	(a) Monthly payroll for nursing staff	£34 245	£35 100	855 A
	(b) Monthly payroll for other staff	£10 425	£12 129	1 704 A
3.	Monthly cost of supplies	£6 015	£8 940	2 925 A
4.	Capital charges	£4 110	£4 274	164 A
	Total direct costs	£54 795	£60 443	5 648 A

First we should explain the meaning of the 'A' placed after each variance. This stands for 'adverse', meaning an unfavourable result, that is, an overspend. If there is an underspend, that would be denoted by 'F' for favourable, although in this example there are no Fs. As you can see immediately, this table seems to show us where our budget has 'gone awry', and even the extent of the overspend.

We immediately note that supplies are overspent by a large amount. This is very useful, and gives us a fairly reliable indication of where to start our investigation. But it is not as refined as it could be. Note that the activity also has a variance. There has been one extra (that is, unbudgeted) patient per day. This in itself, surely, has had some effect on the budget, and would automatically entail more cost. In fact, might not the overspend in money be explained in its entirety by the 'overspend' in activity?

Taking these observations into account we could refine the variance analysis further, by making an allowance for this increase in activity. We do this by means of a 'flexible budget'. This is simply what the budget should have been if the actual level of activity had been foreseen, while the target patient-day expenditure had been achieved. We can calculate the individual flexible items simply by multiplying the actual patient-days by the budgeted patient-day cost, thus:

Flexible budget for June:

1.	Average daily number of patients 26 patient-days = 26×30 = 780		
2.	(a) Monthly payroll for nursing staff	(45.66×780) =	£35 615
	(b) Monthly payroll for other staff	(13.90×780) =	£10 842
3.	Monthly cost of supplies	(8.02×780) =	£6 256
4.	Capital charges	(5.48×780) =	£4 274
	Total direct costs		£56 987

Using these more accurate flexible figures we can now perform a variance analysis. Note that the original budget figures are no longer relevant:

Variance analysis for June:

		Out-turn	Flexible budget	Flexible variance
1.	Average daily number of patients	26	26	—
2.	(a) Monthly payroll for nursing staff	£35 100	£35 615	515 F
	(b) Monthly payroll for other staff	£12 129	£10 842	1 287 A
3.	Monthly cost of supplies	£8 940	£6 256	2 684 A
4.	Capital charges	£4 274	£4 274	—
	Total direct costs	£60 443	£56 987	3 456 A

Now we can see the true extent of the digression from the original budget, and the effect on the separate areas. We note with interest that the nurse payroll, far from being overspent is underspent (hence the F). Somehow the nurses have coped with the extra workload, and have cost less than the budgeted patient-day target. The payroll for other staff is considerably overspent, but the cost of supplies is way beyond the budget. This is where our attention must be urgently directed in the first instance.

Why is there such a massive overspend on supplies? Variance analysis does not tell us the answer to this question, it only directs us to the most critical areas. We must look into the various possibilities. Is it waste? Higher than expected prices? Theft? Maybe a combination of all three. Whatever the cause it should be corrected, so that the budget for the rest of the year can be properly managed.

Even the apparently good result in respect of the nurses should be investigated. The cause of this might not be an acceptable one, for example unpaid overtime (which is not unknown) or a reduction in the quality of care, or a variation in the categories of dependency. And finally, the cause of both a favourable and an adverse variance could be due to the wrong standard, either too low or too high, having been set in the first place; standards should always be scrutinized regularly (as we will be explaining in the next chapter).

If you are wondering how we managed to hit the capital charge so precisely the answer is that the capital charge is, after all, an estimate, and is always a constant total amount, a truly fixed charge, so the amount per patient-day will change automatically with the number of patient-days. If these increase, the charge per patient-day will decrease in inverse proportion, and the total will always be the same.

Marginal costing and pricing

All of the foregoing two chapters has been concerned directly or indirectly with pricing. Getting the price right is a fundamental requirement of any organization. Too high, and the clients will not be forthcoming; too low, and bankruptcy will ensue. As to the price being too high, this is largely a question of what competitors may charge, and at the worst, if you cannot meet their prices (in conjunction with quality) then you go out of business. This is what competition is all about, and is (regrettably or not) at the heart of the new health system of purchasers and providers. As to being too low, we hope that the principles and techniques discussed hitherto will prevent this happening.

There are, however, situations where it might be necessary and possible to reduce prices below what the costing process has indicated. Think about the cost of an appendicetomy as we calculated it in the previous chapter. Here we repeat the calculation for your convenience:

A. Direct fixed costs:
Annual time spent on operations by the surgical team: 1250 hours

			Total	Running total
Annual payroll of the unit			£490 000	£490 000
Capital costs of unit	Depreciation	£50 000		
	Interest	£30 000	£80 000	
Other direct fixed costs		£30 000	£30 000	
Total direct fixed costs				£600 000

1250 hours of clinical activity incur a cost of
£600 000;
therefore 1 hour costs 600 000 / 1250 = £480
An uncomplicated appendicectomy takes

	Total	Running total
1 hour so an appendicectomy costs 480 × 1 =	£480	£480

B. Variable costs   £120   £600
Fluids, anaesthetic materials, disposable
instruments, etc.

C. Ward charge:
Calculated on same principle as A and B:
£85 per patient-day, so ward charge for
this patient:
85 × 5 =   £425   £1 025

D. Indirect fixed costs:

Total general costs for hospital	£10 500 000		
Total patient-days	150 000		

so, cost per patient-day:
10 500 000 / 150 000 = £70

	Total	Running total
and charge to this patient 70 × 5 days =	£350	£1 375
Total cost of uncomplicated appendicectomy		£1 375

Remember that this cost includes a share of all the fixed costs both direct and indirect of the institution. The fixed costs for this unit and for the whole hospital have been shared out in a certain way over all the patients whatever the treatment they have received, and have been or will be paid for. Now, suppose that one more patient needs an appendicectomy; that is, one more patient over and above the many hundreds that have already been included in the budget to arrive at the prices calculated for the various treatments. Should we charge the full £1375 for this extra, or marginal operation?

Well, of course we should, if the patient's purchaser is willing to pay this. But if not, is there a lower figure we could charge without incurring a loss? Look at the pricing table again.

Do we have to charge the £480 for the direct fixed costs? No, because the direct fixed costs of the unit will all have been paid for by the already budgeted patients.

Do we have to charge the £350 for the indirect fixed costs? No, for the same reason; these will already have been paid for by all the budgeted patients of the hospital as a whole.

The only costs that this marginal patient will actually involve us in will be the variable cost in the surgical department, namely £120, and the variable costs incurred in the ward. The variable costs in the ward were reckoned to be £13 per patient-day, which for a nine-day stay amount to £65.

The total of these variable costs is £185, and if we charged only this amount we would suffer no loss; if we charged £186 we would have a surplus of £1 and indeed, whatever we charged over the marginal cost would be pure surplus. So, for example, a charge of half the 'normal' price - say £688 would result in a surplus for this one patient of £503.

To summarize, once the probable throughput of patients has been calculated and prices have been derived from this, then all additional patients can be accepted at whatever lower charge can be negotiated, provided it is no less than the variable costs. Obviously this important procedure depends on the fixed costs being truly fixed – it cannot apply if the number of marginal patients grows so much that it results in an increase in the number of staff, or in any other fixed cost.

Conclusion

We have now come to the end of our brief study of costing and budgeting. We could have discussed such things as incremental budgets, zero-based budgets, case-mix groups (diagnosis-related groups), and cost–benefit analysis.

However we consider that what you have laboured over so far will give you a worthwhile insight into the question of costing and budgeting, probably sufficient for most purposes, and will also be a sound foundation for further study of this topic. Remember, you are needing to grasp the rudiments behind these two important topics so that when the accountants try to bamboozle you, you have the ability to stay with them and argue your case. There will always be people within the organization who have specialist knowledge, and as with every difficult or specialized subject you should not be afraid to seek advice when you need it.

A last word might be that the several demonstrations and illustrations given above might have seemed very complicated and even inappropriate for the real life of a busy hospital, clinic, or social work unit. Well, costing and budgeting (and pricing) have to be tackled difficult or not, but in these marvellous computerized days, complex calculations can be performed by a mere touch on a keyboard.

Further reading

Perrin J (1988) *Resource Management in the NHS*. Chapman & Hall, London.

12

The manager as quality coordinator

In this chapter, we deal with the elements of assuring quality that are the responsibility of the manager; highlights are given of different theories of quality assurance; some of the problems with implementation and motivation are discussed and useful approaches to incorporating quality issues into everyday working practices are given.

Introduction and background

They tried it in America and it didn't work. That's good enough reason for me not to try it here. It'll just be another passing phase that they have thought of to make things that we do already seem more difficult.

We're too busy caring for clients to bother with all these forms and things. Quality is about working with people, not writing about working with people.

Heard anything like that before? If you have had any responsibility for introducing and/or motivating staff to look at quality assurance at work, then the chances are that something along these lines will have been said – probably by more than one person. It is almost a decade now since quality first became an issue within the service sector. However, partly through lack of understanding and also poor management in terms of introducing changes to people, quality assurance as a concept has, to a large extent, got itself a bad name.

The problem, or maybe the greatest strength, of introducing quality as a distinct subject, is that everyone thinks that they already do it. 'Of course we always try and do things the best way possible, are you trying to say that we don't?' The irony is that over tea or coffee, or during the course of everyday working, people moan and moan about the inefficiency of the service.

One of the tricks in getting colleagues to take quality assurance seriously, is to try to get them to make the connection between what they 'do' and what they 'do not' like about the service. If staff feel that their working life can be made easier then they are likely to sign up for something, especially if it relates to improving the level of service available to patients and clients.

What do we mean by quality?

Definitions abound, and it is important that we should try to simplify the language as much as possible. The temptation is always to add jargon to a discipline, because somehow that makes it 'real' or 'professional' and social care settings are no exception. Acronyms and abbreviations abound:

> I went to see the UGM today about TQM in ENT OPD. She said that it would be fine for us to go ahead, but could we wait to hear about ISO 9000 in A&E first as that might have an impact on which way we go.

Even if you understand it, it hardly makes you feel welcome or included in the conversation. As you read through this chapter, make a note of the jargon that will inevitably creep in. Anything that *you* have to look up or think about in the context that it is written, your staff will also need explained to them. Bear this in mind, because it is a useful yardstick by which to judge the topic. It is always hard for us to remember what it is like to get to grips with a subject once we have mastered it ourselves to any extent.

Quality then should be kept simple. Perhaps the best definition is the one given by the Concise Oxford Dictionary which is simplicity itself: 'Degree of excellence'. But this is not going to help to define quality in the workplace. Taking the above definition, it is important to know *whose* concept of excellence we are working towards and to *what* degree that definition of excellence is being practised. Quality as a phenomenon is something that is held in everyone's head (whether or not we always achieve it is a separate issue), but a tacit understanding of what would be considered an acceptable quality of work is present in us all. The problem is that people differ in what they consider to be acceptable quality, as the parameters that we use to judge anything are based on our own unique combination of experience and learning.

The trick is to get people to agree the level of quality and then to make sure that this is not only acceptable, but also desirable. This subtle but very important distinction is exemplified by Case study 12.1.

Case study 12.1

> Consider a nursing home. An acceptable level of quality in terms of nutrition would be a diet that conforms to the norms of calorific intake per day, with an appropriate balance between proteins, carbohydrates and fats. Food should be served three times a day.

> A more desirable level of quality would encompass all of the above, but in addition it would specify temperature of food, presentation of food, choice of menus and a pleasant room in which to take the meals.

Quality is therefore a process and not an absolute. *Agreeing* quality is a process, *achieving* quality is a process and *assuring* quality is a process.

Why should we be interested in quality assurance?

Assuring quality became particularly important during the 1980s in Europe, America and as a result of developments in Japan. Manufacturing industries were the seed bed for this type of pursuit and arguably have an easier path to assuring quality, because they deal with a tangible product that is produced in the same way every time. The things that we wish to assure in the service sector, however, are less tangible – counselling prospective adoptive parents, communicating with someone with a learning disability, for example.

Its transfer from manufacturing to the service sector has been both useful and threatening to different groups. Professional groups in particular have felt threatened by the idea of quality assurance (the term by which any quality activities were first called), as in the past, levels of care and service provision had been their domain. At its most extreme, unconsciously (and sometimes consciously) held values and 'standards' have been perpetuated through education systems, and no one has dared to question 'professional' authority. As an additional safeguard, professional bodies acted as gate-keepers and purveyors of discipline to promote an aura of security and invincibility around professional practice.

The question still remains, however, why should we be interested in assuring quality? There are various possible reasons for this which are broadly political, professional (or perhaps personal), economic and social.

Activity

Make a short note of some of the reasons why you think quality has become so important within the service sector today and what effect these issues might have on why and how we implement a quality strategy. Remember the headings:

Political
Professional
Economic
Social

It is important to work out which reasons you think are driving quality activities, as it will affect not only the perspective that you put on quality, but also your motivation for becoming involved in the first place – remember, if you do not have these things worked out for yourself, you will not be able to convince others and take them along with you as a manager.

It is no coincidence that the introduction of quality assurance to the service sector has become of increasing importance – and ultimately a necessity – as public money has become more scarce and methods of allocating increasingly scarce resources have had to be found. Broadly, the economic and political categories are related to this area. Government has moved more strongly towards the notion of accountability and resource difficulties have meant that people now have to have methods of justifying what they do and how they do it, i.e. value for money and cost-effectiveness.

The professional and social reasons for being involved in quality are probably the two that are more appealing to a workforce. They represent more altruistic reasons, relating to how we see ourselves in society and as professional workers, in an important environment for the welfare of the nation. These reasons relate to why people choose to do their job in a caring profession rather than as an accountant or computer programmer. The recognition of patients and clients as central to work in the caring professions and the increasing importance of their views – both as knowledgeable consumers and interested clients – all feed into the need to be sure of and understand any actions that are taken at work.

Implementing quality management systems at work

Definitions

The way quality matters appear to us at work varies and may be disguised in different ways. Names like total quality management (TQM), continuous quality improvement, quality control, quality assurance, audit, and standards etc. are all bandied around and it would be useful to take a few lines here to look at each one to see what is really meant by the jargon. It could be that you do not need to know what TQM is, but audit and standards are vital to your workplace.

Quality assurance

This is a system designed to make sure that activities are planned in such a way that if they are carried out to an agreed set of standards, then an acceptable level of service will follow according to available resources and timescales. It relies upon a circle of activities (*see* Figure 12.1) which have been variously described by many well-known quality gurus and authors, the most notable of whom by now must be Avedis Donabedian (1966).

Essentially any system of quality assurance must involve an assessment of the current situation, the development of agreed standards by which to move

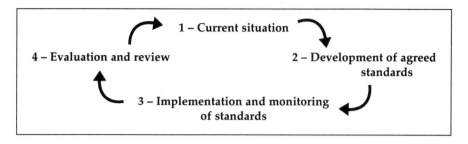

Figure 12.1 The quality assurance cycle.

forwards, implementation of those standards and subsequent monitoring and review which all leads back into the assessment of what will be a future, altered current situation. The procedures involved in this cycle will be discussed in more detail below.

One of the key issues in assuring quality is to see it as an on-going and continuous process. We cannot assure quality one day and assume that it will then hold true for evermore. Continuous quality improvement is therefore one way of looking at quality and making it an on-going process.

Quality control

This is a method for ensuring that the outcome of an intervention reaches an agreed standard every time. It could be used in section 3 of the above cycle, e.g. each time an application is made for housing, then the requisite forms are completed, or each time drugs are dispatched from a pharmacy, accurate stock control and cross checking of the order is carried out.

Audit

A term used to describe any activity in which what happens in reality is checked against pre-ordained criteria or standards – again, section 3 of the cycle. This term originates from professions such as accountancy, but has now grown into a complete branch of quality assurance in its own right. An audit is carried out retrospectively after a procedure or set of activities has been completed, e.g. morbidity and mortality rates after a specified surgical procedure in different operating departments across a region, or waiting times in different out-patient departments, or concurrently during the course of an activity. It is, fundamentally, performance monitoring.

The term audit implies counting somewhere within its domain and this neatly captures the dichotomy between quality and quantity in the field of quality assurance which will be discussed at a later stage in this chapter. Some professions have taken the idea of audit and use it widely, as it is an acceptable notion of quality that produces a number to describe activity.

Medicine in particular emphasizes audit activities, as this fits well with the 'scientific' approach that doctors have to their work.

Total quality management (TQM)

TQM is the concept of an all embracing quality strategy which works for everyone in an organizational setting. It takes as its basic premiss that *no one part* of the organization can produce the best quality on its own, and that there needs to be a clear management commitment in order to pursue the aim of 'total quality'. 'Quality is everybody's responsibility', is one of the key notions in this type of approach.

TQM also takes into account the concept of quality of care plus the quality of service. This is an important distinction within health and social care settings, as it seeks to recognize the need to have good support systems in place in order to be able to produce sound professional service. A residential care home or a community unit cannot provide the best quality of care if the environment is not clean and presentable, or the supplies are not available. Remember, within large organizations *no one* can work *in isolation*.

Standards

Standards form the baseline for much quality assurance activity. *But* the mistake must not be made that standards are the be-all and end-all of working practice. They should *not* be an absolute minimum level of accept-ability, but neither should they prevent people from striving for and achieving a higher level of service.

We have already looked at some of the difficulties in trying to make quality more explicit and tangible, and standards offer one way of moving forward. A standard is defined as an agreed level of performance for a particular population which is achievable, desirable, measurable and observable. If a group of people are brought together who are all concerned with a similar aspect of service provision, and agreement is made about what they wish to write a standard on, then common ground can be established for an absolute level that people will work towards.

ISO9000 (BS5750)

Known as ISO9000 and formerly BS5750, this form of accreditation is a quality management standard awarded by the British Standards Institution (who give kitemarks to electrical equipment for safety standards). It assures a sound system which is designed to reproduce the same quality of service each and every time a product is made or a function is carried out. To gain accreditation, a long process of defining the functions of an organization is undertaken according to the twenty criteria of the British Standard and external auditors are used to check that the system is working. Annual reviews of the system are required during the 3 years of the award in order to maintain accreditation, and the associated expense of the process can be quite high.

ISO9000 originated from the industrial sector and is being adapted to the service sector at present. It has made its mark in the NHS through the process of competitive tendering for support services, where many private sector companies already possess the kitemark, and in order to be able to compete effectively, in-house laundry or cleaning services have had themselves to become accredited. Interestingly however, ISO9000 does not tell you *what* level the quality of the service is, it merely lets you know that the *same* quality will be produced every time.

The move to ISO9000 is spreading into other service sector settings, including those who deliver training courses, an accident and emergency department and also social services departments (*see* Patel, 1994).

Charters and Chartermarks

Charters of all kinds were part of the government's approach to recognizing the needs of the consumer in various services in the UK. There are many different charters that you may have come across, including the Citizen's Charter, the Taxpayer's Charter, the Policing Charter and of course the Patient's Charter to name but a few. The idea of a charter is that a member of the public using the relevant service has a right to expect certain standards of that service and if these are not met then there are channels for complaint and redress.

The difficulty with most of the charters is that they have been written by the relevant profession, based on government guidelines (Cabinet Office, 1991), and not by the consumers. Thus the emphasis that is placed on certain aspects of service provision does not necessarily reflect the true needs of the public. For instance, the Patient's Charter focuses on acute care, waiting times and waiting list figures whereas issues of importance to the public include reasonable standards of clinical skill and care and treatment of individuals as individuals.

Notwithstanding these issues, more recently, Chartermarks have been awarded, which are based on an organization's ability to fulfil all the requirements of the Charter Standard. Broadly the criteria for a Chartermark (which has to be applied for to the Charter Unit) relate to the organization having explicit standards which are monitored and implemented within a unit, taking into account the views of the consumer and having a proper complaints procedure in place. Independent validation of performance against standards is required, plus a 'clear commitment to improving value for money'.

Case Study 12.2 describes a possible scenario that is happening throughout many different units and departments in all care settings. With the advent of purchasing and providing there is the contract culture with built-in monitoring, national standards for the registration and inspection of service facilities, on top of the inherent expectations that you as manager will be able to do everything asked of you when someone else thinks of it.

Activity

What would you do in the situation given in Case study 12.2, and where would you start?

Case study 12.2

> The manager of a family planning clinic (let us call her Lottie) has drawn the short straw. The Trust has got someone in to 'manage quality' and wants representatives from each of the specialities to come along and talk about what they will 'do about quality' within their workplace. The clinical director was not interested and the business manager was far too busy to go along, so Lottie had to respond to the request.
>
> When she got to the meeting she heard people talk about the total quality strategy and aiming for a Chartermark, others sat there not saying very much and she felt totally at a loss to know how to join in. The quality manager spoke about the contracts that they had with the Health Board, as if everyone should know what that meant to them, and made Lottie's toes curl when her clients were described as customers. She was just recovering from the culture shock, when she heard that she was expected to come back to a follow-up meeting in 2 month's time with a set of multidisciplinary standards for her unit, having involved all the staff in the process. Next month's meeting would require a progress report from each person.
>
> 'I want to see a quality framework from each of you that feeds into the Trust's quality strategy. We need to know your customers' views as well as your own and don't forget that the purchasers can change their contracts with us if we are unable to prove that each part of the Trust is providing a valid and quality assured service. I'm here to help if anyone gets stuck, but quality has been with us long enough now for you all to get on with it I'm sure.'
>
> Lottie was dumbstruck and went back to her clinic to try to get some of her colleagues to help out.

Framework for quality assurance

Whose perspective?

As with any potential problem that confronts us, it is best to form some kind of orderly plan or framework within which to work. The quality assurance cycle in Figure 12.1 has a notional starting point which asks for the current situation to be assessed.

What kind of information can this provide? In the first instance if you do not know what you are trying to assess it will patently provide you with nothing. If the above case study is considered, it can be seen that there are different perspectives on this thing called quality which would be a good starting point. Whose perspective do you need to consider? There are the views of your staff and yourself, the requirements of the purchaser, national standards and requirements and the view of the users of your services. At times these views may well be conflicting: your purchaser's priority in terms of efficiency and value for money may well not be what users have in mind (*see* comments under Charters and Chartermarks above) (Figure 12.2).

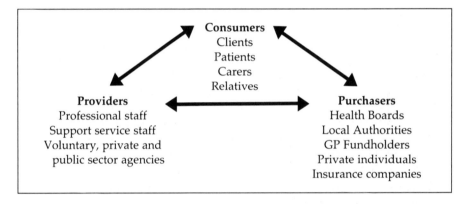

Figure 12.2 Various actors have different perspectives on quality.

If you want to make sure your department or unit is as 'quality assured' as possible therefore, you need to make some decisions about how to knit all these perspectives together. Ask yourself these questions:

- Do you have any professional standards that need to be met?
- What are the mythical standards that are required by your purchaser(s)? Who can tell you that information? (Come to think of it, do you know who your purchaser(s) are and what the purchaser/provider split really means to your capacity to plan and provide your service?)
- What, if any, are the organizational standards required by your parent organization?
- Whose views do you wish to take into account?
- What parts of your service do you think would merit from attention in the first instance?
- What are you key objectives in terms of service provision?

Maxwell's six dimensions of quality

Things are already starting to feel more complicated, but they do not necessarily need to be, as another helpful framework to use is that of Maxwell (1984), who conceived six dimensions of quality. It is always helpful to use a framework to think of quality improvement activities since, as we mentioned earlier, making issues tangible within caring professions is not always easy. By placing your service or any part of it within the following context, it can help you to sort out what it is you should be concentrating on, and also provide you with an outline of how things are actually done.

Maxwell's six dimensions of health care quality are:

1. Access to services
2. Relevance to need (for the whole community)
3. Effectiveness (for individual patients)
4. Equity (fairness)
5. Social acceptability
6. Efficiency and economy.

He went on to describe each of these elements in terms of an accident and emergency service and the analogy is a useful one to use here. Do remember, however, that these *six* dimensions are applicable to most, if not all, service sector settings and there is no reason why they should not be used in, for example, a day centre for the elderly, or any other discreet element of the service. One important point to bear in mind if using these guidelines is that you should remember to view the service from the point of view of the user, as well as the organization.

1. Access to services

Is access to the service limited by time or place, e.g. length of waiting times, geographical location or opening hours.

2. Relevance to need (for the whole community)

Is the service appropriate to the population that it is targeted at. Some assessment of need is required here, against which to assess the provision of the service and its acceptability (supply and demand). In terms of an A&E department this would apply to the availability of major accident facilities, minor trauma treatment, etc.

3. Effectiveness (for individual patients/clients)

Does the service achieve its intended objectives – both in the eyes of the patient and also the staff (technical and personal effectiveness)? To look at this you might consider what equipment and staff are available, record instances of any complications and assess desired outcomes through follow-up assessments.

4. Equity

Is the department providing its services even-handedly despite different cultural or social backgrounds, or physical or mental presentation of patients? There are some elements of access contained within this category, but it also covers issues such as treatment of ethnic minority groups, e.g. available translators, treatment of people with diseases such as HIV or AIDS etc.

5. Social acceptability

Is the service meeting people's expectations? This dimension relates to the environmental and interpersonal aspects of a service. Sticking with the theoretical A&E department, do patients have adequate privacy, what are conditions in the department like, what are standards of communication like – both internally with the patient and other parts of the hospital, and externally with the patient's GP?

6. Efficiency and economy

Are services delivered as efficiently as possible within available resources? Other cost comparisons are needed for this dimension and a working knowledge of what the service can reasonably be expected to provide within the available resources.

Activity

> In relation to your own department or section, think of a single attribute for each of the above categories that would describe your service. Examples might be: the centre will be open between 9 am and 9 pm, 7 days a week (access); the clinic will provide translation services for clients whenever required (equity); the department will consult customers once a year to establish their continuing needs (relevance to need) etc.

Standards

Let us return to Lottie's problem. Where to start? Having done the background work of checking on what standards are expected by other interested parties, the work in the family planning clinic can start. It would be advisable to think of the department in terms of Maxwell's six dimensions. All her staff could get involved in thinking about what issues are included in each of the categories and this would provide a basis on which to devise a set of standards that are desirable for their service. This would satisfy their own need to take a good look at the department and work out what they are really trying to achieve, but would also provide the framework, set in the context of other requirements and regulations, that her quality manager wants for the next meeting.

In devising standards, the form that they take is not, in many ways, the most important issue. Many people get bound up with trying to write a set of perfectly formed and all embracing standards that are then ignored and left alongside the unread policy ledgers on the office shelf. Some people even equate producing a set of standards with quality assurance itself, i.e. 'if we write these, then we will have "done" quality'. Standards are a means to an end and form a very important part of the quality cycle, but they are only one step in the process.

There are many texts which explain the process involved in writing standards and these should be referred to. Ideally, staff should be given some in-house education about this process so that it does not become too time consuming. In this particular example, it has been suggested that Maxwell's six dimensions of quality should be used as a starting point for highlighting topics around which standards can be written. Equally, areas of particular concern or interest to staff can be chosen as a starting point, or feedback from customers and the public could be used to focus the activity.

Indeed, there are many off-the-shelf packages, custom made surveys and in-house sources that can provide information for assessing the areas that should be of concern to an organization or department and therefore the focus of quality activity. In nursing the use of the Phaneuf Nursing Audit (Phaneuf, 1976) or Qualpacs (Wandelt and Ager, 1974) can provide much information on the current quality of care; the use of quality circles within departments or single professional groups have also proved useful and more informal 'quality interest groups' have been used. Patient and client satisfaction surveys are increasing in popularity as well, and highlight potential problem areas that could well be served by inclusion in a quality programme. Any of these techniques (including Maxwell's) can be used to assess the current situation which forms the start of the quality cycle.

In writing standards, there are two approaches which can prove useful. One is to write a statement of fact that relates to the area under consideration and present that in its bald state as the standard. This is the approach that is used in accreditation documents or as part of registration and inspection procedures.

The other approach would be to use standard statements with associated criteria. The best known method for this type of approach is that adapted from the writings of Donabedian (1966). Here a standard statement is made in terms of what is to be achieved and then the component parts are described as criteria in terms of their relation to structure (the tangible conditions needed to support the service, e.g. buildings, personnel, etc.); process (how the service is delivered); and outcomes (the desired effects of the service). In fact Donabedian did not directly link these three components together in the way that we see them as standards today, but this method has been widely utilized, most notably within nursing where the Royal College of Nursing (RCN) carried out extensive work on the introduction of quality concepts to the nursing profession.

The combination of the structures and how they are used are supposed to lead to the outcomes specified, although as we all know in service settings, it is not always possible to guarantee outcomes in the same way as on a production line. Indeed in certain situations in caring professions, it is possible that the outcomes that we desire would happen anyway with or without intervention.

Standards, in whatever form they are written, should relate to only one topic at a time and should be kept as simple as possible. They should be measurable or observable in some way, so that they can be monitored and people can tell whether the standards are being met and if not, then why not. This is *vital*. It relates to what was said above, both in terms of not letting the process of standard definition be the 'be-all and end-all' of the quality process, but also because the quality assurance cycle is just that – a never ending cyclical process.

If continuous improvement and assurance of the quality of a service is not the result of any quality initiative, then there is no point in carrying it out. As we said earlier, you cannot assure quality one day and then hope that it will continue for evermore. It must be possible to actually tell something about the service from being involved in quality and people must *learn* from the experience – either to make sure an action is not repeated in future if the result is undesirable, or to build on good practice and continually seek to find ways to at least maintain it, if not improve it.

Outcomes

It is only right to mention here some of the difficulties that the caring professions have with the concept of defining outcomes. There is a debate as to whether outcomes should be defined merely as what is expected of a specific action, or whether unintended or unexpected effects can also be taken into account. Donabedian (1988) stated that an outcome is 'not simply a measure of health, well-being or any other state. Rather, it is a change in status confidently attributable to antecedent care.'

Enderby (1992) goes on to say that outcome measures, because they must relate directly to a planned intervention, should also relate to a list of expected changes. Thus outcome is specified in goals that are to be achieved. Others however consider the whole issue to be far more complex:

> Patient outcomes are an immensely complex construct. They span the range of results that proceed from (or are assumed to be associated with) the provision of health care services. They are measured both directly and indirectly over differing periods of time and with varying degrees of objectivity, reliability and validity. The desirability of one outcome rather than another in any given clinical situation (e.g. palliation rather than extension of life in the terminally ill

patient) may differ markedly according to the values and preferences of patients, factors that to date are rarely taken into account in outcome studies.

(Lohr, 1988, p.37)

Timing affects the accuracy of an assessment of outcome, since if a treatment or intervention is evaluated immediately on completion the connection between process and outcome can be fairly assumed, e.g. administration of a bronchodilator in asthma to alleviate an acute attack. The longer the time delay, however, the more difficult it becomes to attribute outcome to intervention as confounding variables will have intervened.

The measurement of treatment or interpersonal outcomes is particularly difficult as they are hard to disentangle from the confounding effects of broader societal influences, such as diet, poverty, health related knowledge and attitudes.

It is thus difficult to know whether patient improvement or deterioration is genuinely the result of care provided or a response to concurrent but unrelated change in circumstances.

(Ellis and Whittington, 1993, p.25)

Returning to Donabedian, however, the voice of reason prevails when he states that:

The search for perfection should not blind one to the fact that present techniques, crude as they are, have revealed a range of quality from outstanding to deplorable.

(Donabedian, 1966, p.209)

Any attempt therefore to build on the current state of knowledge in relation to measurement or definition of outcomes must be welcomed.

One final point to make is the difference between outcome and output – important when learning how to use outcome data in planning, delivery and improvement of care. Input and output versus process and outcome can be described as follows.

Input, that is the resources applied, and output, the number of patients treated, are relatively easy to measure; process, that is the the application of resources, and outcome, the long-term effect on patients, are significantly more elusive. The temptation is to relate input to output with a relative neglect of process and outcome.

(Ellis and Whittington, 1993, p.22)

The outcomes of care can thus be stated to be its various effects on patients, assessed by factors such as mortality, health status, level of function, freedom from pain and discomfort, well-being and attitudes to self, health and illness, satisfaction with care, etc. (Ellis and Whittington, 1993). These can be defined as diagnostic outcomes – data required to determine the need for specific care, therapy and prognosis, or therapeutic outcomes – more general aspects of health status (Williamson, 1971).

Monitoring and review

Once you have started to define your service, you will be in a position to undertake some monitoring of the provision of that service. There are various ways that this can be done and once again there are other texts to give more detail about the methods available. It is important though to be able to make decisions about what is most practicable and useful to your situation.

In Lottie's case, she runs a family planning clinic, so there will be a combination of areas that she is interested in and will have approached in terms of standards. She and her colleagues might have written standards in terms of reception of clients, waiting times for clinics (once people are in the building), sterilization of instruments, skill mix of staff in clinics, guidance given for HIV testing, etc. How should she monitor whether the standards are being met?

Activity

Make a short list of ways in which standards could be monitored.

Possibilities include:

- Observation
- Review of documentation
- Questionnaires to staff and clients
- Brief, structured interviews with clients
- Satisfaction surveys
- Review of comments and complaints
- Structured discussion with staff
- Discussion groups
- Log books
- 'Off the shelf' audit packages.

Whichever methods are chosen, the frequency of review and the mechanism must be determined at the outset.

The whole process of quality assurance should be *sensible and planned*, rather than illogical and *ad hoc*.

You will find an in-depth description of each of these methods in Chapter 13 on evaluation. It should help you to decide what way you wish to monitor standards. However, whatever method you choose, do not overdo your monitoring. *Everyone* is monitoring or reviewing their service these days (hotels, shops, British Telecom, etc.) and we all have a degree of 'feedback fatigue'. Be sensible then and put a number of standards together so that they can all be checked at the same time.

Finally, when you have collected any information as part of a monitoring process, then move on to the final stage in the cycle which is to evaluate the results. Were our standards set at the right level? Should we raise them (or perhaps even lower them if there is good reason to think that they can never be reached)? Are there other areas of concern that we should be looking at? What can we learn from this process?

The last point to make in terms of Lottie's problem, is that when she goes back to the meeting equipped with the response to her manager's request, she should be demanding something in return. For Lottie's clinic to really feel that quality is of importance, then they need some kind of evidence that the Trust itself is quality orientated. Just reading a mission statement in the monthly newsletter *Trust Yourself*, or knowing that there is someone in post as a 'quality manager' will not convince anyone that things have changed. The organization needs to show its staff that it is committed to quality through an open policy on upward communication (*see* Chapter 8), managing by walking about (*see* Chapter 2), and by taking positive results from other units' and clinics' quality initiatives and making them available to all.

Finally, the Trust's own quality strategy should be known and understood by all staff, so that they feel committed to it and so that if anyone is asked they can explain what the benefits of this type of approach are. (Interestingly, this is one of the checks that is made by the external auditors for ISO9000. Staff are asked at random if they are aware of the department's quality strategy and what it means in terms of their job.) If, as a manager, you do not feel that you are getting support for the demands that are being placed upon you and your staff, then this has to be pointed out. Trying to motivate others to undertake a token gesture is more counterproductive than constructive.

Potential benefits of taking part in a quality assurance initiative

Going through the process of describing your service at a macro or micro level – for instance you might be in charge of a series of facilities, each of which could undertake an analysis of themselves using Maxwell's dimensions – also means that you start to justify what you do and how you do it. In terms of trying to achieve extra funding for a new resource or increased staffing for a particular service, resource allocators are far more likely to listen to people who have a well thought out case, rather than someone who turns round and says something like 'well of course we need another crèche assistant, the service has changed beyond all recognition since it started'. Why? In response to what? How has it changed and by how much? Statements and standards of service can help to clarify the position and through monitoring and review you, as a manager, should know far more about your service than just gut reactions and unsubstantiated facts.

The single most important aim in a quality assured organization, is to *maintain and improve the level of service* that is available to clients, customers, patients, users, the public. The level of job satisfaction, the potential savings in effort, time and money and a greater agreement about the actual point of the service are all secondary to this. If anyone needed convincing of the necessity to make the effort to get involved in quality activities, then they should consider this as motivation.

Conclusion

In total quality management terms, it has already been stated that quality is everyone's responsibility. The biggest benefit that can be gained from this type of approach, however, is for different parts of the organization to learn that they are interdependent. The level of tribalism within any hierarchical organization is quite marked and whilst these often artificial boundaries and patterns of communication are maintained, then a true quality culture cannot be promoted. Cooperation and taking responsibility for what you do are the building blocks of a quality organization and are positive attributes to which anyone can aspire.

References

Cabinet Office (1991) *The Citizen's Charter. Raising the Standard.* Cmd 1599. HMSO, London.

Donabedian A (1966) Evaluating the quality of medical care. In Schulberg HC and Baker F (eds) (1979) *Program Evaluation in the Health Fields,* pp. 186–218. Human Services Press.

Donabedian A (1988) Quality assessment and assurance: unity of purpose, diversity of means. *Inquiry* 25, 173–92.

Ellis R (ed.) (1988) *Professional Competence and Quality Assurance in the Caring Professions,* Chapman & Hall, London.

Ellis R and Whittington D (1993) *Quality Assurance in Health Care: A Handbook.* Edward Arnold, London.

Enderby P (1992) Outcome measures in speech therapy: impairment, disability, handicap and distress. *Health Trends* 24(2), 61–4

Lohr K N (1988) Outcome measurement: concepts and questions. *Inquiry* 25, 37–50

Maxwell R (1984) Perspectives in NHS management. Quality assessment in health. *British Medical Journal* 288 (12 May), 1470–2

Phaneuf M C (1976) *The Nursing Audit - Self Regulation in Nursing Practice.* Appleton Century Crofts, New York.

Wandelt M A and Ager J W (1974) *Quality Patient Care Scale.* Appleton Century Crofts, New York.

Williamson J W (1971) Evaluating quality of patient care. A strategy relating outcome and process assessment. *Journal of the American Medical Association* 218(4), 564–9.

Further reading

Bond S and Thomas L H (1991) Issues in measuring outcomes of nursing. *Journal of Advanced Nursing* 16, 1492–502.

Donabedian A (1986) Criteria and standards for quality assessment and monitoring. *Quality Review Bulletin* 12, 99–108.

Hogg C and Cowl J (1994) Different strokes. *Health Service Journal*, 12 May, pp. 28–29.

Kitson A L (1987) Raising standards of clinical practice - the fundamental issue of effective nursing practice. *Journal of Advanced Nursing* 12, 321–9.

Koch H (1993) Buying and selling high-quality health care. In Spurgeon P (ed.) *The New Face of the NHS*, pp. 146 – 59. Longman, Harlow.

Patel A (1994) Quality assurance (BS5750) in Social Services Departments. *International Journal of Healthcare Quality Assurance* 7(2) 26–32.

13

The manager as evaluator

In this chapter you will learn to think about how to evaluate different parts of your work; look at how to set up an evaluation and consider the pros and cons of various different approaches to information collection that are open to you.

What is meant by evaluation?

We have already pointed out that there are many demands on your time as a manager: people asking you to provide them with information, to motivate your staff, to ensure a good quality of service is provided, to absorb the latest changes in policy and structure within the organization and so on. Most of the time, work feels like 'fire-fighting', i.e. you react to things as they happen and deal with them as and when they occur, rather than being able to look ahead and foresee events. The ideal, of course, would be to have some control over things. This book is one attempt at helping you to deal with all these competing demands by looking at issues such as time management and team building etc.

But even when changes are well planned, how do you know whether they are worth while or effective? Think about other areas for which you have responsibility such as quality (*see* Chapter 12), communications (Chapter 8) or the introduction of a new rota system. How can you tell if the actions that have been taken have produced the required outcomes, or indeed, any effects at all? How can you assure your purchasers that you are giving them value for money? Various answers to this thorny problem exist, and they all relate to the topic of evaluation.

Evaluation can be defined as: 'The process of determining the merit or worth or value of something; or the product of that process' (Scriven, 1981, p. 53) Evaluation is about the process of making decisions. These might be at different levels – for instance, practitioners wish to know whether they are giving the right care, whilst managers wish to know the relative merits of the care in terms of efficiency and value for money. Essentially though, people need to be able to make a reasoned choice about what their service does and how this is provided.

The timing of an evaluation can be important since you will get different information depending when you take a look at the issue that you have in mind. If you look at a new innovation do you want to evaluate it whilst it is still developing, or do you want to wait until it is established? Would you want to speak to students during a course, or would it be easier or better to wait until the end of the course? The decision about timing will partly depend on what type of information you require and also when you have the time and the opportunity to actually undertake the work.

If, for instance, you are setting up a new project or trying a different style of management with your team, it is useful to think about what might help an evaluation right at the outset. The best planned evaluations start with the beginning of something new, since you can be routinely collecting pieces of information that will be useful in the future and certain interviews or other enquiries can be made over a period of time to see exactly how things are developing.

Monitoring

At times, you might not need to look at something in a questioning way. It may be enough to simply know what is happening – say on an activity basis when numbers of visits or clients, per day or month is adequate. This type of knowledge is gained through *monitoring* a service and you will often come across the two terms – monitoring and evaluation – together.

Monitoring is an on-going process that is normally carried out routinely and usually takes quite a structured form. If you fill in monthly returns for any aspect of your job or track your staff hours or shifts, then this will provide you with monitoring information. It lets you keep an eye on things in a simple way and may provide you with useful data if and when you come to evaluate any aspect of your work.

Imagine that you run an employment support service and want to know about numbers and types of clients seen over a monthly period. A simple form with appropriately labelled columns will enable you to tick off each person as you see them, record when you saw them, how long for, what they came for, e.g. education, employment or training advice, and what follow-up action is necessary – if any. At the end of each month figures can be collated and total numbers in different categories can be easily put together for the annual report. None of this information tells you about the quality of the service or if the service is what clients actually want, but it provides you with sound data on how your time is spent and with whom etc. You have monitored and not evaluated.

Most of this chapter is spent discussing evaluation as it is the more complex process of the two. Do not neglect monitoring as part of your work though and remember to approach it in a sensible and well thought out way. It is as easy to collect useless information as it is to collect information that is useful – but we shall discuss this in more detail later in the chapter.

How do evaluation and quality fit together?

You should be recognizing some of the issues that came up in quality assurance, and it is true that evaluation and quality have many things in common. There is a major difference between the two topics however, which relates to the fact that in pursuit of quality, the aim is to set standards and assure them in practice. In contrast, evaluation is a process of investigation and not affirmation; it may look at the component parts of a system or process, but then decisions are made about the value of that system or process, from which it is possible to deduce the standard that currently exists.

Quality and evaluation can be related, however, if we consider the quality cycle and in particular, the monitoring phase where actual practice is looked at against predetermined criteria or standards (*see* Chapter 12). (Do not confuse the term 'monitoring phase' with the concept of more global monitoring mentioned above. The monitoring part of the quality cycle is the time when activity in terms of standards is checked against reality. Monitoring as an on-going process is something more consistent as we have described.) The results of any evaluation will help us know to what extent we are meeting the standards which have been set, and should also say where and how things could be improved to meet or improve the standard that is being aimed at. Without knowing what is happening in reality, quality assurance cannot exist, because you do not have the evidence to prove to anybody what you are trying to assure them of.

Whose responsibility is it?

Organizational evaluation

Evaluation can happen in different ways within the work environment and not all the responsibility will lie with you for 'determining the merit or value of something'. At times, your organization will seek to evaluate some new innovation or existing practice. You will be expected to cooperate in this process and as manager, to encourage your colleagues to do the same. Certain issues can arise around these larger projects however, which put people off the concept of evaluation – or any critical appraisal of their situation.

Activity

Think of a management led survey, audit or 'fact finding' mission that you have been asked to take part in:

- How much information were you required to provide?
- Did you ever receive a copy of the finished report?
- Was your department informed of the results relating to them?
- Did you even hear whether the survey was finished or not?
- As a manager, were you invited along to a presentation of results?

Various points to be made in this chapter will help you to learn how important it is to carry out any information gathering exercise properly, but at this stage just remember that when you finish a piece of evaluative work, always let the people involved in providing you with information know about the results. Even more importantly, let them know what actions you are going to take based on these results – even if it is that things are going well and will therefore stay the same. It is natural for people to get annoyed and disillusioned when they have contributed to something and have not been told anything about the outcome of that process. We become suspicious and resentful and will certainly be dubious about participating when the next audit or survey comes along (as it inevitably will) if we feel that we have been taken for granted in the past.

Activity

Other types of evaluation occur at the organizational level as well. Take a few moments to think of the type of statutory inspections or accreditations that your work area contributes to.

For instance in Scotland, if you work in a nursing home or residential home of some sort, then you will be inspected by your local social work department and/or health board inspection teams. The Scottish Hospitals Advisory Service goes out to all hospitals where people live and the Mental Welfare Commission visits any establishment where there are people being detained under any part of the Mental Health Act (Scotland). Mental Illness Specific Grant projects are monitored and evaluated by the social work department and ultimately the Scottish Office. You might work in an organization or department that has ISO9000 registration. The point being made here is that there are external agencies who also evaluate your work and you should be aware of these processes and what they mean to you and your team. Remember though, the same principle also applies in relation to external inspection or visits – you should make sure you receive feedback. If someone else has done the work, you might as well benefit from it.

Departmental evaluation

In terms of your own responsibility for evaluating your work practices, there are various forms that this might take. Not all of them necessarily involve you in a lot of work – or even any real effort at all. Take the example of everyday contact with colleagues. There will be times when you will be trying to introduce something, or solve a problem at work that someone else has already tackled. By talking to colleagues about their experiences, you will form an opinion about the innovation (probably backed up by others in the organization) and will decide then whether to proceed with it, modify it or drop it. You have, essentially, made an evaluation of your position on the basis of which you have taken a reasoned decision. Colleagues have some knowledge of your particular area of work, but more importantly they will see things from a different perspective.

This is important in the process of evaluation, as you need to pick up information from a variety of sources or using a variety of methods, in order to corroborate the evidence that you are gathering. (If all this sounds a bit like detective work, do not worry, as you are not going to 'try a case', but in a sense you are following clues to try to understand whatever situation you are evaluating.) Contact with colleagues is a very important process, because it stops us 're-inventing the wheel'. If someone else has tried something, it will give an indication – even at a subjective level – about whether the change or innovation has worked. Only through a systematic evaluation, even on a small scale, can you hope to make these judgements. It is a truism that many things in large, bureaucratic organizations continue to exist simply because no one has questioned their worth – because it exists, it must be all right.

How to plan and implement an evaluation

It is very important when you are planning any discreet piece of work to have a logical plan of action, so that the work is well thought out before it is attempted. Much time is wasted through bad planning and ill thought through projects. They will not give you the useful information that you require and will annoy those involved, as they will see yet another piece of work coming to nothing with no actions being taken at the end.

In setting up an evaluation, the following questions should be considered at the outset:

- Why is the evaluation necessary?
- Who is to carry it out?
- Are all the staff committed to the process?
- What are the criteria for evaluation?
- Who is the evaluation for, i.e. what audience(s)?
- How are the data to be collected?

- When is the best time to undertake the evaluation and how long is it to take?
- How will it be presented and followed up?

Case study 13.1

Lottie, the family planning clinic manager we met on page 152, has more problems. She is getting some feedback from clients about a new counselling service that has been introduced. Some comments are good, but others indicate that there might b˒ some problems. In addition, the staff running the service are expressing some doubts about its effectiveness and they want to know how long it is going to continue under its 'trial period'.

The service was started originally because there seemed to be a demand and someone had read about a similar service on offer elsewhere in the country. There had been some discussion between staff about how the service should be set up, but mostly it had been made to fit in around current patterns of work.

How can Lottie evaluate the service? What does she need to consider in relation to the service to give her a full picture on which to base a decision about its future provision?

Activity

What would you do in response to the problem set out in Case study 13.1? Think about the list of questions posed above and jot down some pointers that will help to plan a successful evaluation of this particular issue.

Let us go through the stages of planning the evaluation one by one:

- *Why is the evaluation necessary?* Lottie needs to be able to show whether the new service is really worth while so that it can be continued, modified or stopped in the future. She also needs to know whether it is meeting the needs of her clients, as well as fulfilling its organizational responsibilities in terms of value for money.
- *What are the criteria for the evaluation?*
  - Are the clients satisfied?
  - Is the service being well used?
  - Can it be improved in any way?
  - Is the service as efficient as possible?
- *How are the data to be collected?* There are many ways to collect information – not only through questionnaires or interviews. In the next section we

will consider different methods of collecting data as putting out a questionnaire is not always the answer.

- *Who is to carry it out?* Lottie has two members of staff who are interested in the project and would like to take the opportunity to improve their skills in this area.
- *Are all the staff committed to the process?* Lottie will introduce the evaluation to colleagues at the next staff meeting and discuss the reasons for wanting to collect the information and then take suggestions from her staff about how they think the study could be undertaken. It is important to involve staff from the outset, especially as any changes to the service and any feedback from service users will need to be acted upon by the department's staff.
- *Who is the evaluation for?* The evaluation is for internal use only in this instance, although Lottie will be able to use some of the findings in her next annual report when she is compiling a profile of the service – how they have looked at client needs and assured that a high quality of service has been maintained.
- *When is the best time to undertake the evaluation and how long is it to take?* There are no other studies planned for the near future and Lottie checks with other staff in the department to make sure that they are not planning anything that would conflict with this piece of work. It can therefore be carried out now and should be completed within 6 weeks.
- *How will it be presented and followed up?* A short written report will be prepared so that the results will be available on file for future reference. Feedback will also take place at the next available staff meeting after the end of the project.

So, Lottie has considered all the questions before starting the evaluation. Not all the answers would be so straightforward all the time, but you can see the idea behind asking yourself a logical sequence of questions before you leap into what is a fairly major piece of work on top of the provision of your normal service.

Methods for monitoring and evaluating

In this section, we shall consider various methods that are open to you for monitoring and evaluation within your work setting. These are also mentioned briefly in Chapter 12 on quality and standards, and the application of different methods for collecting information could be useful to you in many aspects of your work.

It is important to stress at this point that this is *not* an instructional text on methodology. What we are trying to do is to open your eyes to the possibilities that you have and what some of the drawbacks and benefits are in each case. Too often, you can read textbooks which tell you how to do something, but fail to let you know when, or why, you should be doing it.

The possibilities that we shall consider represent a broad range of methodologies that could be considered when planning any evaluation and could be used with either staff or patients/clients. Methods include:

- Structured/semi-structured questionnaires
- Structured/semi-structured interviews
- Discussion or focus groups with staff/clients
- Review of documentation and existing data
- Logs or diaries
- Observation
- 'Off-the-shelf' audit packages
- Satisfaction surveys
- Review of comments and complaints.

If you look at the above list – which is not necessarily exhaustive in terms of all available methods – you will see that there are different kinds of data collection techniques. Some of the methods will provide you with what is called 'qualitative' data, e.g. observation and focus groups, whilst others will give you 'quantitative' data, e.g. structured questionnaires. There are many differences between the two types of data and you should be aware of what kind of information it is that you wish to collect. Table 13.1 illustrates some of the differences between qualitative and quantitative to give you an idea of how and when each could/should be used.

Table 13.1 Qualitative or quantitative?

Quantitative	*Qualitative*
Considers 'how many?'	'Softer' approach
Provides generalizable results	Looks at perceptions and experience
Open to statistical analysis	Looks at 'why and how?'
Systematic/predetermined approach	Is an adaptable approach according to
Sometimes seen as 'scientific'	what you find
Provides a snapshot, or longitudinal	Seeks patterns of response
information	Useful for sensitive topics

Qualitative information will give you an idea of people's impressions and can be used to understand people's experience of the service. Remember, if someone has the perception that your service is slow or unhelpful, it does not matter whether you agree or not, something makes the recipient feel that way and it may be that you will need to change something. Some people might say - why should we change the service on the basis of one person's complaint or bad experience? In each case, you would need to consider the 'evidence' that has been presented to you through the information that you have collected and make a sensible decision about the severity or acceptability of the data before you decide to make wholesale alterations. As with most things, there is no hard or fast rule, since your information might vary from professional misconduct to complaints about the colour of the paint in the department.

Quantitative information, which tells us how much and how many, is useful for monitoring activity or expenditure etc. Knowing how often equipment is used, or how many clients are being seen, or how much money is spent on dressings by different district nurses for similar patients can all bring valuable insights into your service. Often a combination of both kinds of information will be what is needed, to enable you to understand your service more accurately.

How to choose what methods to use

Whatever methods you decide to use for monitoring or evaluation, always check that the knowledge and the expertise are available in relation to that particular method. In addition, consider what seems most appropriate for the study that you want to do. Do not go and construct an enormous questionnaire when talking to people would be more appropriate, and do not spend money on an off-the-shelf package when a few well thought out questions could get you the information that you want. Your biggest problems in relation to collecting information will probably be expertise in putting good questions together and finding staff time to carry out the study. Knowledge of the different techniques might mitigate against some of them being used, but courses are available to learn how to collect and utilize data – and in large departments the chances are that someone knows how to construct a questionnaire or review documentation etc.

Some thoughts on collecting information

In recent years, everyone from the local supermarket, to your bank and any hotel want to 'know your views about our service'. In other words people are beginning to suffer from feedback fatigue. If you decide to monitor or evaluate situations within your work, be creative and choose different methods so that people are not bored by the prospect of filling out yet another form or providing you with a set of answers. Keep people's attention and make sure that any questions you ask are understandable, relevant and jargon free. If you design a questionnaire or interview for use, always try it out on a few guinea-pigs first (metaphorically speaking!). It is worth the effort and saves a lot of misunderstanding in the long run. What might seem obvious to you can be gibberish to the next person.

Another factor in choosing how to collect information concerns the ability of people to provide you with the information you want. Do not ask people questions in English if their first language is Urdu or Chinese. Do not ask people to fill out forms if they have difficulty in seeing or writing. It may sound obvious, but it will affect the amount and the quality of the information that you get back. Some people will prefer to speak to you on their own and others would rather be in a small group or with someone else. Be sensitive to people's needs: if you are going to observe an interaction make sure people know that you are there. In all cases, always obtain the consent of the individuals – whether clients, patients or staff – to having their views taken and recorded.

Certain factors inhibit people from giving useful responses and if you consider the kind of setting that you are working in, then that can be an additional stress factor for respondents. People are ill or in need of support when they see us professionally, they have not chosen to come along unlike visiting a museum or theatre. The most common, and in a sense the most difficult problem that faces us, is knowing when people are telling you what they really think and when they are telling you what they think you want to know. The so-called satisfaction surveys of clients and patients that are carried out on a grand scale are a good example of this. Most people when they are asked about a service will tell you that it is 'fine'. They will say either that they are not qualified to judge or that they cannot criticize constructively.

Why should this be? For many patients or clients, there is the fear factor. 'If I criticize this service, then it might get taken away from me/people might not like me/I might get penalized next time I come back/people will ignore me if I say negative things.' For staff, unless you have a very open and trusting department, people can be dubious about career prospects or working relationships if they are seen to criticize. It is easier therefore to give the questioner the information that you think they want. This gets the service nowhere – unless you want good publicity.

There can also be problems with distractions or pressures of time. An easy way to get clients or patients to answer questions is when they are a captive audience within your department, i.e. when they are waiting to be seen. But here people are so concerned about missing their names being called that they cannot really concentrate on your questions. If you visit people at home, it is difficult for them to say 'no' to you if you ask them to participate. Then there is the television on in the corner, the dog snapping at your heels or children rushing in and out – all the normal things to contend with in a client's home! None of these factors will help the person to concentrate on what you are asking.

Finally, before you are put off asking people questions altogether, there are difficulties with memory. Our perspective on time tends to blur situations in our memories and we can confuse one situation with another. We also 'telescope' time so that we think things happened fairly recently when in fact they happened a longer time ago. For accurate recall therefore it is best to ask people about recent experiences if at all possible (no more than 6 months ago).

Methods of collecting information

Each methodology has its own strengths and weaknesses and there are many texts which will give you greater guidance on how to utilize each technique (Quinn Patton, 1990; Oppenheim, 1992; Connor, 1993). It would be useful to consider here, however, some of the more obvious factors in relation to the most popular methods.

Questionnaires

The first thing to be aware of is that questionnaires are by no means as easy to construct as they seem and they should certainly not be the first option. You cannot just jot down a few questions and leave it at that. It is tremendously difficult to put together a coherent set of questions that will actually get you the information that you want.

Activity

Look at the following two examples and think what is unclear or unhelpful about them:

Example 1
1) Did you find the department:
a) Clean ☐   b) Unclean ☐
c) Tidy   ☐   d) Untidy ☐
e) Noisy ☐   f) Quiet ☐

Example 2
2a) Tell me, how helpful were the staff to you today during your interview?

2b) In the future, would you rather than we were open between 9am and 10.30am, or 2pm and 3.30pm?

The first example does not tell you how many boxes you are allowed to tick (one or more?). What if you thought the place was unfriendly to children or difficult to find? The second example contains leading questions – if you ask how helpful the staff were, then a respondent is less likely to be negative. In addition, the opening times have obviously been decided by the staff prior to consulting the public – what if neither time is acceptable, for instance if I work? There is no room for disagreement. These are very simple examples, but they are easily repeatable when trying to ask sensible questions of people.

So, when are questionnaires useful? If you wish to get responses from a large number of people then this is one way of doing that in a relatively cost-effective way. In addition you are not dependent on everyone being available on the day that you happen to have free for interviewing or observing. Make sure that everyone gets a clear set of instructions with their form and knows what to do with it when they have filled it in. You must be able to assure people that what information they are giving is confidential and that they will not be identified through what they have said. Questionnaires are also useful for getting quantitative and qualitative information at the same time. Provide people with a list of choices about your service but always put in a category for 'other comments' or 'any further comments' (*see* Figure 13.1).

SA–Strongly Agree A–Agree N–Neither agree nor disagree D–Disagree
SD–Strongly Disagree

4. Communication with colleagues					

	SA	A	N	D	SD
4.1 My immediate manager keeps me informed of plans/developments					
4.2 He/she communicates what is expected of me at work					
4.3 I feel that I have someone to talk to when I need help with something related to my work					
4.4 My immediate colleagues/team members communicate adequately with each other					
4.5 Development of devolved management will assist me in communicating with colleagues					

Any further comments on questions in section 4?

Figure 13.1 Example questionnaire.

In this example there are definite choices offered for most of the question, but there is a space at the end for further comments. Another point, look at question 4.5 – remember what was said about jargon? To be able to answer this question you would need to know what devolved management was, so target your questions carefully. Look at each part of the question and you can see that each one only asks about one aspect of communication with colleagues. One of the easiest things to do in a questionnaire is mix up more than one issue in a question. For example,

'Did your support worker explain the process of applying for benefits to you and did this help clarify things for you?'
Yes ☐   No ☐   Don't know ☐

Well, yes, she explained things to me but I am no better off for the explanation! How do I answer?

One final thought is that if you do decide to use questionnaires then make sure that whenever you ask people's opinions you are not only asking the questions that you want answers to. What do we mean by that? Basically, in constructing any interview or questionnaire form, it is easy to bias questions to get the information that you want rather than what the person really thinks. It is also sometimes easier not to ask about some things altogether, to limit the person's choice by not asking them about certain topics, so that they do not tell you about the awkward aspects of your job.

Activity

How could Lottie have used questionnaires? List one or two ways in which you think questionnaires might help her current situation.

Realistically, the best use of questionnaires in Lottie's situation would be to produce something that is short and easy to complete for all users of the service. It could ask basic questions about accessibility of the service, reasons for choosing to use it, what changes they would like to make to it if any, how often they have attended, whether it has met their expectations, etc.

The main message for questionnaires then, is think carefully before you decide when to use them and be careful in putting the questions together. Consider the checklist in Figure 13.2.

Interviews/discussion groups

This can be a better way to get information back from patients and clients since it is simpler for them to take part and you can explain anything that they do not understand as you go along. You can also get more information through interviews than you will get from any written responses. Interviews need to be designed with the same care as questionnaires however, although there is room for some leeway since the interviewer can help to explain unusual terms etc.

If you want it to be, an interview can be as structured as a questionnaire. Have you ever been involved in a market research interview? Someone asks you what you think about the reliability of British Telecom payphones and asks you to rate your answer on a scale of 1–10, where 1 is poor and 10 is excellent; or they ask you 'which of the following washing powders do you use regularly?' Both of these are really spoken questionnaires as they do not give you room to make up your own response. Frequently, interviews will be what is called 'semi-structured', i.e. you ask a question but allow the respondent to tell you what they think is a relevant answer in relation to the central topic.

Does anyone in-house have expertise in designing questionnaires?
↓
Always pilot a questionnaire before using it
↓
Do not ask leading questions
↓
Use a combination of open and closed questions
↓
Design the form with ease of analysis in mind – do not make it too long or complicated
↓
Only ask one thing at a time in each question
↓
Each individual should receive his/her own questionnaire
↓
Always set a timescale for the return of the form
↓
Give clear instructions about how to complete the form
↓
Let people know where to return the form to, in confidence

Figure 13.2 Questionnaire checklist.

If the interview is to be even more loosely structured and you see a small number of people at the same time, then this becomes a discussion group. Here you will set a topic for consideration, e.g. transport facilities to local day centres, and then the group will freewheel around the subject until all ideas and contributions are exhausted. This type of session can be difficult to record as more than one person may be speaking at the same time. It can be useful therefore to have someone in as a scribe whilst you concentrate on the actual interaction.

Other types of interview (which can also be structured, semi-structured or unstructured) include telephone interviews and 'mobile' interviews. The former are, as you would expect, carried out over the telephone in order to save time in meeting with people. The latter concern interviews where you actually talk to someone whilst they are walking/travelling around. This can serve two purposes: it can save people time again and it also allows you to observe people at their work whilst actually talking to them.

Accurate recording of interviews

In talking about making an accurate record of interviews, we do not literally mean a tape recording, but any kind of record that captures the essence of the interview. Tape recording ensures that you take the whole interview away with you, but this then needs transcribing and probably contains some parts that were not particularly relevant to the questions. Making notes as you go along, then, is the other most likely option and as with most things you get more practised at this over time. Make sure whatever you write is legible and as comprehensive as possible, since even after a short space of time, one interview will get confused with another in your mind and you will lose the detail quite easily. It is vital to capture the responses at the time and not promise yourself that you will check your notes at the end of the session after you have completed three or four interviews.

Carrying out interviews

In order to use interviews for evaluation or research purposes, professional staff have to be given some training first. Though most health and social care staff use interviews as part of their everyday work pattern, they are trained to carry out a staff/client interview, not interviewer/interviewee. The main difference lies in the fact that as a member of staff your response to a professional interview will be guided by the advice that you wish to give (or may be asked for), or you will be giving your opinion. You do not engage the client in the same way for a research interview. This type of interview will always be at your request, you should not give your opinion on any of the questions as this could lead the interviewee in their response and every interviewee must be asked all the questions contained in the schedule. You cannot gauge feedback if everyone was not given a chance to respond to the same questions. Having carried out literally hundreds of interviews, we can safely say that there must be hundreds of people who think that we agree with what *they* think, since you nod and look interested in order to get them to expand on their theory of communication, client rights, the state of the health service today etc. Remember – bite your tongue and do not argue with the respondent. If there is something that you would like to debate with someone, then do it at the end of the interview once you have finished recording what they say.

When planning to interview people, think about whether they would be happier to be seen alone or with others. Some respondents will feel threatened by the formal atmosphere of an interview, and gain moral support from being with their peers – particularly staff. In terms of patients or clients, the likelihood of seeing more than one person at once would really only be in a discussion group, where personal opinions can be aired but potentially confidential information would not be required.

There are two major *drawbacks* to interviewing: the *time* that it takes and the fact that you only collect the information that the *interviewee remembers* when you are in a room with them. Have you ever been speaking to someone and walked out of the room, only to remember the three things you really wanted to say? Apart from anything else, by asking people questions you will be prompting them to think of things that they might not otherwise have considered and they will mull over this even after you have gone. You can potentially lose valuable information.

One way round this is to let people see the questions before you ask them, since they can then give the topics some thought before seeing you. Another way is to be available after the event either in person or over the phone so that you can be contacted with the 'extra' information that people forgot on the day. In reality very few people avail themselves of either form of help, but it may be worth it even for one person's 'extra' recollection.

In relation to the new service at the clinic, interviews will probably form a good part of Lottie's evaluation. But do they all need to be on a one-to-one basis?

Activity

Who would you interview and what questions would you ask? Note down some of the reasons for interviewing in this case.

Lottie is dealing with a potentially sensitive service. Interviews will help to deal with this. Staff providing the service could be seen as a group. Time can be spent discussing the pros and cons of the current arrangements and as with any group format, the ideas that one person has will probably 'spark' others off to think more expansively about the service than if you had seen each of them individually. It might also be useful to interview the clinic manager who is responsible for the timetabling of services. She would have thoughts on usage and accessibility that others may not have noticed.

Finally, there are some responsibilities that interviewers must note. They need to locate the person that they wish to interview, find a mutually convenient time, have some space to carry out the interview, be able to record the responses accurately and legibly (most important!) and agree a time limit at the outset. In other words when thinking of interviews, consider the checklist in Figure 13.3.

Review of existing information

One of the most important lessons to learn in any walk of life is:

DON'T RE-INVENT THE WHEEL!

Why go out and try to collect some information that already exists within the system? More and more information is collected these days in the name of administration/management information systems and for some of the things that you might wish to know, the data will already be there. Each month you must complete forms detailing such things as patient or client contacts, staff sickness rates, holidays, and many of you may also have to provide financial returns as well. All of this information when looked at over time will tell you a story. Patterns or trends will emerge in the figures/information and whilst it will not necessarily tell you why things are happening, it will tell you what

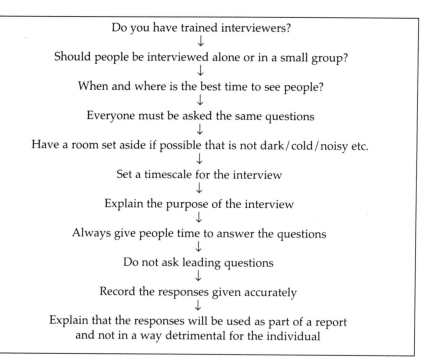

Figure 13.3 Interview checklist.

was actually happening in activity terms. Did staff sickness alter at all when you introduced that new pattern of working? Have the overtime budget figures altered since you got another part time member of staff in to cover the evenings?

Think of Lottie's problem with the new service at the clinic. One of the first things that she should do is to see how the numbers of clients have changed over time. Have they built up, is there a regular pattern of contacts, is one counsellor busier than another, is one time of day more popular than another? As she begins to study the information that will have been collected through the appointments book, a picture of this new service will begin to emerge and she will not have had to do anything other than consult existing records to get to the information.

One very specific way to use existing information to inform you about your service is to look at the nature and number of the suggestions or complaints. These form a very tangible feedback loop for your service and will not only indicate to you what you should be concerned about, but also when something has been sorted out. To take a very common example for hospitals, there are always numerous complaints about parking facilities (there are never enough spaces). If, over a period of say two years the percentage number of complaints drops after you have tried to rectify the situation, then it is one way of knowing that the action that you have taken has had some effect. The additional benefit of tracking complaints is that you will also be dealing with clients and their perception of the service will be helped by the fact that you are dealing with their concerns.

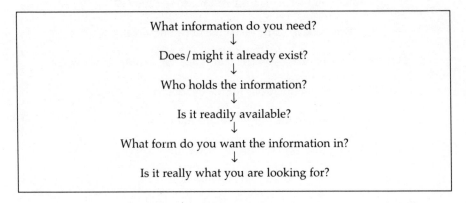

What information do you need?
↓
Does/might it already exist?
↓
Who holds the information?
↓
Is it readily available?
↓
What form do you want the information in?
↓
Is it really what you are looking for?

Figure 13.4 Reviewing information checklist.

Figure 13.4 gives a checklist of steps to follow in reviewing information.

Logs or diaries

At times, you will want to collect some quite detailed information that helps you to 'get inside' the service as it is provided, or to try to get staff to interpret their work in more depth. For either of these instances, the use of diaries or logs can be of benefit.

A diary is something that you may ask a patient or client to use: 'Fill in your experience of the service over the coming week, looking in particular at the way people talk to you, the level of comfort that you have and the amount of choice you are given in what happens to you.'

A log is slightly more structured in that you will ask people to make a record of certain types of instances only, for example when staff encounter difficult situations at work. This leads to detail about one topic rather than their whole experience of being at work.

Advantages of logs

One of the great advantages of either diaries or logs, is that you capture the information relating to any given situation as and when it happens. This gets over the problem of what tricks our memories can play, allows for a recording to be made over a period of time (therefore you do not have to remember everything at once) and also allows situations or details to be recorded that people were not aware of until they came across them. Imagine the amount of information that you could potentially get back from these sources. It will be very unstructured, particularly in diary form, but the depth of the description should be quite illuminating. Of course, it can only be used with people who are well enough or literate enough to be able to undertake the task, and as such will preclude some people.

A piece of research into how we relate to ourselves what we do was carried out by Donald Schön (1991) and helps to illustrate the value of this type of recording. He put forward the idea of 'theories of action' and 'theories in use'. If we were to ask you how you would react in a given situation – say if someone had an aggressive outburst in your department – you could detail what your actions would probably be. If we were to come and watch you dealing with this situation however, we would probably observe something if not very different, then at least slightly different. That does not mean that you lied when you described your actions to us, but it indicates that reality often differs from theory. How we would *like* to see ourselves is not necessarily how we are.

Using training logs

Imagine that you wish to discuss someone's possible training needs at their annual appraisal. They will have their own ideas about time management, professional skills, counselling courses, etc. that they would like to attend. You may have other insights to offer as their manager when you have noticed deficits in their required skills. So between you, you can identify most of the obvious needs of that member of staff. But what about the more hidden difficulties that the person might have, and how do you know what to prioritize for them in terms of any input you might recommend them for?

If you get the person to fill in a training log over a period of say a fortnight or a month at work, then you will begin to get an insight into both of these problems. By asking them to record situations when they felt that they could not complete their work to the best of their ability or satisfaction (do not say 'when they have done something wrong'!), they can begin to appraise why that should have been the case and also give some thought to what the possible solution might be. The act of making a record catches everyday situations that people find themselves in where they might not have realized that they had a training need. It also produces a very personalized record for any staff member. It cannot, however, catch up with situations where people do not perceive they have a need, which is particularly difficult in terms of attitudinal problems.

The use of logs and diaries is summarized in a checklist given in Figure 13.5.

Observation

Observation aims to collect more in-depth information in the same way that the log or diary does. When you observe people or situations at work, you

Do you want a running commentary on an experience?
↓
Do you need to capture information as events happen?
↓
Is the respondent in a position to keep a record?
↓
Give explicit, straightforward instructions for recording
↓
Structure the record where possible to capture relevant information
↓
Keep the recording period to a realistic timescale
↓
Make sure you are able to cope with the volume / depth of information that you will get back

Figure 13.5 Logs and diaries checklist.

may be said to be either participant or non-participant. These terms are self explanatory, i.e. you either observe by being part of a situation, or observe at a distance and not as part of the interaction. By observing people as they actually carry out their work, once again you can see how people actually do things rather than listen to what they or others have to say. You will already spend a lot of your time unconsciously observing everyday situations, the difference in using it as an evaluation technique is that you will make a record of the observation and check things off against predetermined criteria. You are also going into a situation knowing that you are there to observe and will therefore be prepared to sift through all the images that you come across in order to interpret them according to your criteria. Do not go and sit in an out-patients' clinic waiting area to try to observe the skill of your staff at answering telephones for instance.

Observation is a difficult methodology to choose, particularly if you are known to the people involved. Everyone gets self conscious if they think they are being 'watched', although the situation tends to normalize after the passage of time. It could be argued that, as with any investigative methods, merely looking at something will have an effect on how it works – the Heisenberg Uncertainty Principle or the Hawthorn Effect are well-known terms to describe this phenomenon. Observation can make this more apparent simply because of the selfconsciousness of human nature. It does not negate observation as a sound way of gaining useful information however. What better way to find out what it is like to be a client than to go and use the service, or at least follow someone's 'career' through the role of being a patient or client?

Some of the nursing quality instruments, such as Qualpacs, use observation as one of the main data collection techniques and it is important in any situation such as this to show the staff being observed what will be involved. In this way, it is possible to work towards a feeling of trust in an observation situation, since each party will be aware of what exactly is happening. It can also help those being observed to understand what is happening and to feel that by taking part in the event they have the chance to contribute to the enquiry.

Why do you need to observe something?
↓
Be certain what you will be looking for
↓
Dedicate sufficient time to the exercise
↓
Practice observing and recording before you do the 'real' observation
↓
Repeat the exercise on more than one occasion to get a true picture
↓
Always explain to people what you are doing

Figure 13.6 Observation checklist.

To sum up, observation can be a challenge and as with all the methods it takes some skill to carry it out well. The richness of the information that can be gained, however, from watching things as they actually happen can be worth the effort and with some forethought some of the obstacles could be overcome (Figure 13.6).

Off-the-shelf packages

There are numerous commercial, off-the-shelf packages available for monitoring, measuring, evaluating or examining situations. This is not the place to list them, particularly as the number and versions available is constantly changing. How many times though, assuming you can afford to buy them in the first place, are they 'not quite right for my situation'? It is also possible that you are meant to buy the expertise to make them work as well as the documents themselves; an option that is not open to most middle managers.

The cautionary tale here then is to make sure that the package will do exactly what you want it to rather than you doing exactly what the package wants you to! Sometimes someone offers you what seems to be an easy solution and it is very tempting to take it. However, what may be a time saving blessing in the short term will not necessarily be so economical in the long term. Figure 13.7 gives a checklist for the use of off-the-shelf packages.

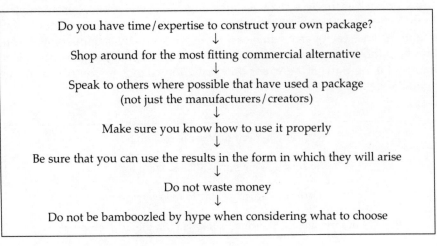

Do you have time / expertise to construct your own package?
↓
Shop around for the most fitting commercial alternative
↓
Speak to others where possible that have used a package
(not just the manufacturers / creators)
↓
Make sure you know how to use it properly
↓
Be sure that you can use the results in the form in which they will arise
↓
Do not waste money
↓
Do not be bamboozled by hype when considering what to choose

Figure 13.7 Off-the-shelf packages checklist.

What to do with information that you have collected?

One vital rule in any kind of data collection exercise is: DO NOT COLLECT MORE DATA THAN YOU CAN HANDLE.

It may sound contrary after all the above advice, but actually collecting information is not the most difficult thing to do. It is all too easy on finishing a study, to find yourself confronted with mounds of paper that just make you want to panic because of the enormity of the task! If you are trying to complete this whilst holding down your normal job, then do think about this stage in the process when planning what methods to use.

Making use of visual means to assist understanding

Whenever you are considering presenting information in report form you should consider how visual means such pie charts, tables and graphs might complement and enhance your text. We use the word complement advisedly since you do not want to present just a whole mass of tables or graphs – your readers can easily become irritated and may not complete their reading. Try to set illustrations and text together on the page, resist the temptation to pull all the visuals into an appendix. Many readers will not bother turning over the pages.

Suppose that Lottie wants to present information on the age profile of the women who are making use of the family planning clinic in any one year. She could present this information as shown in Table 13.2. However she might want to illustrate the bunching effects of those seeking advice who are aged between 22 and 28. She could present this as a graph as shown in Figure 13.8.

Table 13.2 Age profile of women using the family planning clinic.

Age range	Numbers attending
16–18 years	26
18–20	32
20–22	38
22–24	50
24–26	56
26–28	65
28–30	59
30–35	49
35–40	35
40–45	22
Over 45	5

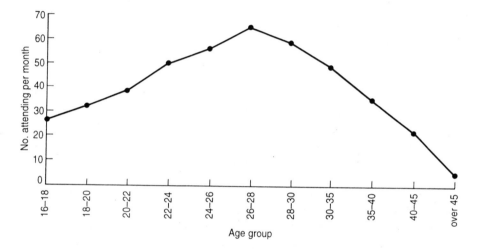

Figure 13.8 Number of clients attending the clinic, presented as a graph.

On the other hand she might find that presenting this information in pie chart form would make the material easier to see at a glance. A good many reports now include pie charts. The development of special software on PCs now makes this much easier to do. There are various ways in which such pie charts can be drawn. Figure 13.9 shows the 'ordinary' pie chart with the size of the various segments matching the numbers on the table.

However if you wish to highlight one particular segment of the pie chart – for instance the number of women aged 16–18 coming for advice to the clinic – then you can 'float' this particular 'piece' to illustrate its special/different nature (*see* Figure 13.10).

If you are not going to use these visual devices but prefer to rely on tables then remember that it is well worth your while experimenting either on your PC or simply with ruler and pencil to see what would be the most effective

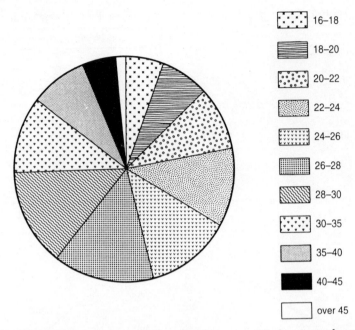

16–18	
18–20	
20–22	
22–24	
24–26	
26–28	
28–30	
30–35	
35–40	
40–45	
over 45	

Figure 13.9 Number of clients attending the clinic, presented as a pie chart.

method of laying out the numbers. Always tell your reader if you are rounding up to the nearest whole number.

Set out your data in a visually attractive manner. You will generally find that it is easier to read information in vertical columns rather than horizontal ones. For instance compare Tables 13.3 and 13.4. In general it is easier to spot variations when the data are set out in vertical layout rather than horizontal formation.

What you want from your efforts is concise, understandable and above all useful information. A long and rambling list of what people said or who does what is not enough. In the case of an evaluation, simply regurgitating figures or phrases will not suffice. Remember, you are trying to 'determine the merit or value of something'. This means that you are making judgements and interpreting the data that you have collected. It is worth remembering these points before you even start to collect information because the time and expertise you have to give to this part of any evaluation or study should determine how you collect your information.

Analysing information

Analysing information is yet another skilled task and one that needs to be allocated an adequate amount of time. This part of an evaluation however may be one that you are most familiar with, since your duties as a manager

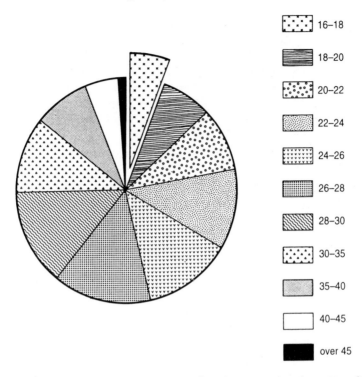

░░░	16–18
▤	18–20
░░░	20–22
▒	22–24
▽▽▽	24–26
▦	26–28
◩	28–30
░░░	30–35
▒	35–40
☐	40–45
■	over 45

Figure 13.10 Number of clients attending the clinic, presented as a modified pie chart.

Table 13.3

Year	1986	1987	1988	1989	1990	1991	1992	1993	1994
Visits to clinic	201	213	229	312	355	388	442	478	389
Phone calls	1290	1398	1467	1578	1681	1656	1734	1674	1867
Referral from GP	121	178	198	178	129	198	325	298	341

Table 13.4

Year	Visits	Phone calls	Referrals from GP
1986	201	1290	121
1987	213	1398	178
1988	229	1467	198
1989	312	1578	178
1990	355	1681	129
1991	388	1656	198
1992	442	1734	325
1993	478	1674	298
1994	389	1867	341

will probably require skills needed to interpret information and draw conclusions. The important part of monitoring or evaluating is to prepare some kind of action document from any analysis that you undertake. This does not always mean that a lengthy written report has to be put together, although if you wish to share your results with others, then this may be necessary. You may want to produce action sheets for particular staff members, pull out parts of the result to send to *your* managers to show them how well you are all doing or simply discuss things with people.

So, how can you let people know what you have done? You have finished the work, and prepared a record of it. If you have used staff or patients and clients to gather information from, do not forget to tell them that the study is finished. As we said earlier, too many studies simply disappear into the mists of time and the depths of the organization. Then, if you have made any recommendations or drawn any conclusions, discuss these with people and choose something that you can get to work on straight away. It is important to take immediate action following an evaluation to show people that you are committed to the study and wish to use it to everyone's benefit in the workplace.

Whatever type of analysis that you decide to undertake, it is possible that you will use a computer at some stage of the process (or if you are not using one yourself then you may be working with a secretary who will be). It is important to remember, if this is the case, that you have to be aware of people's rights under the Data Protection Act (1984). The development of the Act came from a growing public concern about the amount of information that was being held about each of us on various organizational computer systems. As someone who may be recording information on a computer, you have to be open about the records that you keep and follow certain guidelines (Data Protection Registrar, 1989). Where a computer is used to merely type up a report, then the Act does not apply, but if you are recording and processing information in *any* way (even by keeping it to add to in the future), then you must register with the Data Protection Registrar. The information that is relevant to the Act relates to anything that can identify a living individual. So even if you do not type in someone's name against a set of responses, a reference to their grade and working location, or disability and home locality may prove to be enough to distinguish them from the rest of the respondents.

Conclusion

At different times in your career as a manager, you will be asked to look critically at the services under your charge. You need to know how you can at least set about doing this and what is realistically possible given the constraints within which you work. Always make any study manageable but worthwhile.

At times you should consider a monitoring exercise and sometimes you will need a more in-depth evaluation of services. The information contained here should enable you to make decisions about how either of these processes could best be undertaken. Your skill, as with anything that you practise, will grow over time and you should consider improving the expertise of some of your staff in data collection techniques. The more in-house experience that there is in designing and implementing and completing a study, the more chance you have of producing a worthwhile and useful product.

References

Connor Anne (1993) *Monitoring and Evaluation made Easy. A Handbook for Voluntary Organisations.* HMSO, Edinburgh.

Data Protection Registrar (1989) *The Guideline Series and Guidance Notes, 1–8.* Office of the Data Protection Registrar, Cheshire.

Oppenheim A N (1992) *Questionnaire Design, Interviewing and Attitude Measurement.* Pinter Publishers, London.

Quinn Patton Michael (1990) *Qualitative Evaluation and Research Methods*, 2nd edn. Sage, California.

Schön D A (1991) *The Reflective Practitioner*, 2nd edn. Avebury, Burgess Hill.

Scriven M (1981) *Evaluation Thesaurus*, 3rd edn. Edgepress, California.

Further reading

Shropshire Health Authority (1992) *Getting to the Core. A practical guide to understanding users' experience in the Health Service.* Shropshire Health Authority in Conjunction with University of Birmingham.

Whiteley S J (1989) The Construction of an Evaluation Model for use in Conjunction with Continuing Education Courses in the Nursing Profession. Unpublished PhD thesis, Queen Margaret College, Edinburgh.

14

Making the best of your staff

In this chapter we examine recruitment and selection of staff, job and person specifications, induction processes, coaching and mentoring, staff development motivation, training and appraisal.

We have already said that the bulk of all costs involved in health and social care are in staff salaries and wages with attendant costs in terms of National Insurance, pension contributions, etc. Any manager must be aware of this fact of life and seek to make the very best of human capital. All too often managers say that their staff are important and that they deserve to be given time and yet in practice, through the pressures of work, fail to spend much time with their staff at all. Ask yourself how much time you are spending with your staff? This chapter is deliberately entitled 'Making the best of your staff' to highlight this important management function and to provide you with ideas to further your 'investment' with staff.

Let us trace the various stages of our contact with a member of staff. Not all these stages will apply equally to all readers, however as devolved management increases then it is likely that more managers will be involved in these processes.

Recruitment and selection

Some of you will be spending a great deal of your time on this work, others will only be rarely involved. Here then is a brief survey of this area.

We will start with a hole – a vacancy. Someone has resigned, retired or a gap has been identified. If someone has left then the first and increasingly obvious question to ask is: do we need to replace this post? Other questions that we might ask are: Does the job need to change to meet the changing needs and objectives of the department/unit? What kind of skill mix do we want now and in the future? The person we wish to recruit will thus be seen in terms of a range of skills held by members of the team/unit/department etc. and we will need to look at complementary skills within the team.

Where managers have been very satisfied with the performance of the previous post holder, there is a tendency to try to find an identikit person to replace him or her. This can be very restrictive. Consider as well the fact that the previous job holder may have altered the job very much to suit his or her particular interests. Unless we think through the nature of this vacancy then we may be swayed by such a person's idiosyncratic contribution.

Job description

A job description should describe the various tasks and responsibilities which comprise the job. It should also suggest the various weightings in terms of the responsibilities and where the post holder should concentrate his or her efforts.

The problem with many job descriptions is that they sit in desks and are seldom, if ever, dusted off and looked at. All job descriptions should be subject to regular review.

Job descriptions are important in a number of ways:

- they provide a clear indication of what is expected of a member of staff;
- they form the basis of recruitment and selection, i.e. in drawing up an advertisement;
- they provide the basis for assessing training needs; and
- they provide a baseline for appraisal.

Here is a brief checklist for you to use in making up a job description:

- *Job details.* This should include the job title, the current grade (if applicable), the name of the section or unit, and the location of the post.
- *Purpose of the job.* This should provide a concise statement as to why the job should exist.
- *Scope of the job.* This should cover information concerning the scope of the job in as factual a way as possible, e.g. responsible to Mrs Smith for computer maintenance.
- *How the job fits into the care service.* Who is the line manager to whom this person should report?
- *Knowledge, skills and experience required.* This should summarize the main knowledge, skills, attitudes and experience required to perform the job to a competent level. If the post requires particular professional/technical qualifications then these should be indicated.
- *Key results areas.* These are statements concerning the 'end results' required of a job. Ideally they provide an indication of outcomes, achievements and standards rather than a list of duties and tasks. The main characteristics of key results areas are that they:
  - represent the key outputs of the job;

– are worded in terms that emphasize action that leads to an end result;

– use specific wording rather than vague statements;

– provide the basis for a measurement of work against standards; and

– can help in identifying training needs.

Identifying key results areas can often prove the most demanding part of a job description. However in this form they can be reviewed more easily in the light of changes in health and social care. They provide the line manager and post holder with objectives to aim at. Normally one should consider around five key areas and certainly no more than ten. We will be revisiting key results areas later in this chapter when we examine appraisals.

● *Communications and working relationships.* This describes the various people within the organization with whom the job holder needs to have contact. It should also specify the *type* of communication and *its purpose* in relation to the section/department etc.

Job description agreement

For existing jobs with their job holders in post it is good practice for the manager to discuss and agree that the job description is indeed accurate, comprehensive and clear. An appraisal interview usually starts with this clarification; it provides a useful opportunity to dispel any role blur.

Sources of information in drawing up your job description

Useful information sources include:

● existing job descriptions;
● current job holders' experience;
● outside contacts, i.e. what they do in another hospital, care centre;
● results from appraisal and job reviews; and
● departmental plans, organizational plans, national standards, etc.

Compiling a person specification

When you have examined the job description carefully and consulted various colleagues, then it is helpful to think about the necessary categories for the person specification. This is a way of helping you when either making a selection for a new post, replacing someone in an existing post, or when considering a clarification or setting of role for an existing staff member (this could come about as a result of an appraisal interview). The following categories are not intended to be a set format, simply guides – use them as a basis for your needs.

Physical considerations

Are there any aspects of the job about which special qualifications should be specified in terms of being able to work under particular conditions? Are there any adaptations to the description that could be used to make it more possible to employ a disabled person?

Education and training

Are there any particular requirements specified (apart from the obvious professional and technical ones), such as a recent qualification in HIV control)?

Experience

Does this need to be directly relevant or could similar kinds of experience in a different environment (non-health or social care) be considered an advantage? There are various points to be considered here: length of time spent doing a job may not always be so important as range and variety of experience.

Specialist skills and knowledge

Some skills can be assessed at interview (computing, keyboard) but the more complex ones such as aspects of management ability can only be judged on the basis of previous record. If we are looking at internal candidates, the question may be: how quickly can this person be trained up to a satisfactory skill level?

Personality and disposition

This is a very difficult area. We may be looking for someone for the receptionist post at a health centre who is 'outgoing, friendly and gets on with people'. The difficulty is in assessing these traits. If we are using existing staff, a redeployment for instance, then it is quite possible that we and others in a supervisory position will have formed some impressions as to the person's personality etc. However, as we know, some people may not show their true personality if managed in a particular way, and their outgoing, friendly nature may not blossom.

If we are selecting someone new then this area is difficult to assess and most prone to bias.

Special circumstances

This only forms a part of the person specification where it is *relevant* to the job, e.g. being away from home for long periods, working at weekends, etc.

Great care must be taken when asking these questions, otherwise overt discrimination may occur if they appear to be about the *person* and not the particular *job* in question.

Legal aspects in recruitment and selection

The law in the UK

The Sex Discrimination Act 1975 and the Race Relations Act 1976 make it illegal for any employer (or employer's representative) to discriminate unfairly against an individual on the basis of his or her sex, marriage, colour, nationality, race, ethnic and national origin. The Employment of Disabled Persons Act 1958 requires employers to recruit people with disabilities.

If you are using this text outside the UK you will need to be familiar with your own country's laws. Check whether your organization has a policy with regard to these matters. For example, here is an example taken from a UK educational organization.

> The X organization confirms its commitment to a comprehensible policy of equal opportunities in employment in which individuals are selected, promoted and otherwise treated on the basis of their relevant merits and abilities. No job applicants or employee should receive less than favourable treatment on any grounds not relevant to good employment practice.

Direct discrimination consists of treating a person on grounds of race, sex, marital status, etc. less favourably than others would be in similar situations. This type of discrimination is the easiest to spot; however what is more difficult is *indirect discrimination*. This consists of applying a condition or prerequirement for a job which, although applied to all, is such that the proportion of one group (for example, women) who can comply with it is considerably smaller than the proportion of other groups.

For example, setting unnecessarily high 'physical strength' standards in terms of selection criteria for a job could indirectly discriminate against women. Indirect discrimination can occur when recruiting only through uninvited, 'on spec', letters of application or CVs, since only particularly confident people may apply.

Positive (affirmative) action

This is a process of actively encouraging people from a particular group – race or gender, disabled, etc. to apply for particular posts if they have been or currently are under-represented in that area of work. For example:

> The X organization has no women currently working in the field of... and would particular welcome applications from suitably qualified and experienced women.

The law requires that appointments are made on the basis of merit. Applicants must be treated *equally* when it comes to the actual selection process. This is a crucial point.

Induction

Having prepared the job description and person specification and interviewed and selected the best person with due regard to the various laws that apply, the next step in 'making the best of your staff' is induction.

There is some evidence from surveys conducted by the Institute of Personnel Management over the years, that the quality of induction can have a very important effect on how staff later feel about the organization they have joined. A poor induction can easily give the impression that senior staff do not bother that much with staff and that newcomers are expected to 'sink or swim'.

At the same time there is a danger that if we make the induction process too restrictive and prescriptive it may stifle individual initiative and creative thinking. We must take care that staff coming fresh into their posts are asked of their opinions and encouraged to ask, 'Why does this have to be done like this? Couldn't there be a better way?' So often an induction process and the attitudes of existing staff prevent newcomers asking such questions; they are made to feel that such comments are cheeky and that as a newcomer they should keep quiet and not express their true feelings and doubts. Yet if our organizations are to change such newcomers are the very people we should as managers be asking, since they do not carry any of the baggage lugged around by those who work for a long time in one organization.

It is a difficult balance: on the one hand we must provide some comfort for our new staff: they must feel welcomed and they need to be reassured as to their duties and fully informed as to the various administrative procedures; on the other hand we do not want mere clones of the existing workforce to emerge.

Activity

Consider your induction into your present job. What were the positive aspects? Were there any aspects that might have been improved?

We mentioned in Chapter 2 that one of the problems for staff in times of rapid change is that of role blur. One very important function of induction is to make sure that the new member of staff is fully briefed as to his or her various responsibilities.

If you have an induction procedure it is always well worth reviewing it. It is a very useful exercise to ask those who have recently experienced 'your' induction their views as to what they felt was positive and what could have been improved.

Mentoring

This can be part of an induction process. A new member of staff is teamed up with someone who 'knows the ropes' and can act as a mentor. This relationship does not have to occur just during induction, mentoring can be a key aspect of staff development.

A mentor is a person who has a responsibility for a colleague not in line management terms, appraising and supervising, but in being available to assist, ready to listen and advise. Many organizations have taken mentoring very seriously. They realize that there are many occasions at work when a member of staff needs reassurance and advice and that this is often more comfortably expressed in an informal way rather than using the more formal channels of supervisor or manager. The difference between this and just being good friends is that mentoring is set up deliberately. In many ways it is similar to coaching (discussed below): if it is going to happen then it has to be planned for, staff have to be informed as to what the expectations are, some awareness of training needs to be laid on, and the 'ground rules' of the system have to be explored and clarified.

Basically everyone in the organization, no matter how junior or senior, needs a mentor – someone who will be there when needed. Senior staff are often the ones under most stress and they can most certainly benefit from having a mentor. For example, in a hospital one ward is widely recognized for its excellence of patient care; that ward sister is being used to mentor other sisters and charge nurses elsewhere in the same hospital – that is, she is used as a sounding board, advice centre and source of ideas.

Here are some other examples of what mentors can do:

- listen carefully and question when a colleague plans a tricky course of action;
- run through an appraisal interview before the colleague goes for the real thing with his or her boss;
- act as devil's advocate and ask awkward questions at a rehearsal of a presentation;
- compare notes on such things as filing systems, approaches to time management, the running of meetings, etc.

Coaching

The relationship established between those involved in mentoring is similar in many ways to that needed between a coach and the person being coached. Coaching is in essence a form of delegation, as we saw in Chapter 2. It is a form of planned delegation from one person to another.

These days, with the need to upgrade skills and train staff to be able to cope with change (and with budgets for training which do not expand very rapidly), the development of coaching is increasingly important.

Case study 14.1

> A member of staff is required to use a new piece of software which will speed up access to patients' records. The member of staff has had no experience of this software. The alternatives are to:
>
> - read the manual and get on with it;
> - read the manual and seek help via the telephone with the software company;
> - go on a training course run by another hospital;
> - find someone in the hospital who has worked with a similar software package and ask him or her to coach.

Case study 14.2

> A member of staff in the kitchen of a residential home is uncertain how to test the smoke alarms. She had been shown by the company who had installed them but that was some months ago and she has forgotten. Again she could read the manual (complicated) etc. But how much better if she had someone who could spare a few minutes and actually do some coaching on the complications of the system.

The two examples in Case studies 14.1 and 14.2 illustrate the range of coaching that is possible. Coaching is a form of staff training and development in which one person demonstrates, teaches, guides, and generally takes some measure of responsibility for a colleague's increased awareness, skills, competence, knowledge, etc.

It is *training* in that the staff member is able to work more efficiently and effectively. It is *staff development* in that the person being coached and the person doing the coaching are both increasing their skills and abilities and gaining in confidence.

Coaching should not be seen as a cheap alternative to other kinds of training – especially sending people away on courses. It is complementary to other training. As we have said with mentoring, coaching is not something that will just happen. You as a manager need to actively pursue it.

There is probably a great deal of unofficial coaching already going on within your organization, that is to say staff with more skills are helping those with less. Managers have to guide it, set up the system, discuss with those involved the 'ground rules' and provide some awareness training. Sometimes you as manager will be doing the coaching but mostly you will simply facilitate it. If you are both manager and coach you will often have to distinguish between the two roles. As a manager you might want to take a more directive approach at any given moment, reminding the person as to agreed standards, but your role as coach must always be collaborative.

Creating the right atmosphere for coaching

Coaches must create and develop a working relationship which encourages individuals to improve their own working practices. We have seen in terms of motivation theory and practice that simply *telling* people what to do only achieves a short term improvement. Coaching is based on collaboration and effective two way communication.

Qualities of a good coach

The qualities displayed by a good coach include:

- a skill or understanding which is of high standard;
- a willingness to pass on this skill and understanding;
- a need to be committed to the other person's success;
- an enthusiasm for high standards and belief that these are attainable;
- a consistency of approach;
- a sensible use of control – encouraging the person coached to think for himself/herself and encouraging the person to experiment with techniques/approaches and to take some risks (but controlled).

A good coach tries to operate on an 'adult to adult' approach in Transactional Analysis terms. It is so easy for the coaching relationship to turn into parent (telling) and child (accepting). The adult relationship means that the coach will be prepared to let the person try things out and therefore take some risks. Coaching and mentoring are very much part of motivating your staff – truly making the best of them – to which we now turn.

Motivation

Motivation comes from the Latin *'movere'* to move, and thus involves getting action.

In general terms, there are three kinds of strategies that we can use to motivate people. These are summed up as:

- the push approach or the use of sticks to beat people into action;
- the pull approach or the use of rewards and incentives to encourage people into action; and
- the achievement approach or encouraging people to do things because they want to.

Push approaches

These are predominately based on the principle that the way to get action is to evoke fear in the individual through the use of threats and potential punishment. They are often characterized by the phrase: 'You had better do this or else . . . !'

The problem with the push approach is that it tends to get a 'push back' response from the individual which can take the form of childlike behaviour (in TA terms, the 'child' reacting to the 'parent') or, in extreme cases, subversive behaviour. Nevertheless, some managers still think that they can only get the performance they want by pushing.

Pull approaches

These are based on the idea that people are looking for external rewards (carrots) for the effort they put in to achieve the action required. Such rewards can be relatively light, e.g. thank you, an acknowledgement from the boss that a job has been well done, a salary review or a bonus. Like the push approaches they tend to be external to the individual although they are based on a more constructive and positive philosophy of management. The problem with the pull approach is that it tends to be short lived, so that, for example, the carrot gets eaten and more carrots are demanded to get action in the future. Nevertheless these are commonly used to try to motivate people in schemes such as performance related pay.

Achievement approaches

These are based on the principle that people are most highly motivated by those things that they want to do. For example, most people do not need to be motivated to take a holiday, pursue a hobby or develop their career. People are motivated to do these things because they have developed a personal responsibility towards the goal which they are seeking to achieve.

If you pause for a moment to reflect on what motivates you in your job, you will probably mention job satisfaction or a job well done, or a feeling of doing something worthwhile, e.g. a grateful patient or a satisfied client. This sense of achievement and recognition for undertaking work which is in itself a worthwhile activity is likely to be a strong source (for you) of motivation, it is what gets you up in the morning to face whatever challenges and problems the day may bring. To put it crudely, although you want to be paid a reasonable return for your efforts, you are not really in it for the money.

These brief introductions to different approaches have to be put into a context of individual difference. There are many books and theories written specifically on the subject of work motivation, but here we are going to discuss just one approach: Maslow's theory of human needs.

Maslow's theory of human needs

At any given point in your life, some needs may be more important to you than others and seeking to satisfy these needs may be the main source of motivation for you. In his work on needs, Maslow (1954)identified five levels or grades of needs in human beings which help us to understand what may be motivating an individual at any given point. He saw these needs as forming a hierarchy from lower to higher order needs and they are presented below with examples of how work *may* help to meet them:

- *Basic needs*: These are mainly physiological, such as food and water to satisfy hunger and thirst. In an industrial society, most people do not have to concern themselves with these needs because they are so readily met. At work, money is likely to be the main means of satisfying these needs.
- *Safety and security needs*: These mainly provide protection from your enemies and provide a secure future but they also include warmth and clothing i.e. protection from the elements. Work related examples would be pension schemes, a degree of certainty that your job is secure, and, again, money, which helps to satisfy some of these needs, i.e. it can provide the means for you to have a home or save for the future.
- *Social and affection needs*: These are mainly concerned with our need to be with and interact with other people – to be part of a group and accepted within it. At work, there are many opportunities to interact with others – colleagues, patients and clients – and to be a member of a team, which can be very important for some people. Many other writers have stressed the importance of the social group at work and changing social groupings can have a demotivating effect.
- *Ego and self esteem*: This is mainly about recognition of your worth as a person, having self respect and the feeling that you are accomplishing something worth while in your life. Work can provide many satisfactions of these needs, for example through recognition that you are doing a socially worthwhile job, through being held in high regard by your colleagues and employer, and through tangible means such as job titles, office space and company cars. Equally, we can experience being treated in a way that discounts our hard work and efforts and the consequential lowering of self esteem that this can bring.
- *Self actualization*: This is the achievement of your potential in terms of your skills and talents as a human being. At work, for some, the challenges of the changes and developments taking place have been experienced in this way – they have felt that their talents and skills have been stretched to the full and they have achieved things at work which previously they would have thought unlikely. Promotion can be experienced in this way with the new job making demands and requiring the development of new skills and knowledge. Maslow suggested that the realization of all our potential as human beings was a rare or 'peak'

experience and that this would not occur for many. He also considered that once experienced and mastered, new challenges and developments would need to be faced for this to again become a source of motivation. It is clearly important for some people that they be given new challenges in their jobs and faced with demanding targets on a regular basis.

Although a little dated, Maslow's work throws some light on what matters to an individual. He argued that seeking to satisfy needs involved moving through the different levels outlined above and that lower order needs had to be met before higher order needs became important to the individual. For instance, if your job is threatened by some changes (security needs not satisfied) then you are likely to be motivated towards satisfying that need and higher order needs may be of little relevance until this has happened.

Relating this to work settings, we can at least recognize that people may be satisfying different needs by being in employment. For some, money may be perceived as a very important source of motivation because it is the basis on which the lower order needs are met and at their stage of life these needs are more uncertain. For others, work is an opportunity to meet other people and to enjoy social interaction even when a job might be very routine and boring. And finally, for a few people, work is the means whereby all their talents and skills are fully realized (self actualization).

Techniques

In the light of this discussion on motivation, what techniques are available to managers to help motivate staff?

Leadership style

The particular style of leadership you use will have a direct influence on staff. If you tend to have to 'push' staff, i.e. using threats and pressure relatively consistently, then your style will probably often produce a 'push-back' effect as outlined above. On the other hand, if you tend to involve people in the decision-making process, e.g. by consulting before a decision is made and encouraging ideas and commitment to the final outcome, you are more likely to evoke personal responsibility on the part of the other person and arrive at a decision that they want to make work. As a leader you need to identify what is important to your team members and seek to balance satisfaction of these needs with the demands of the task itself.

Objective setting

This becomes, among other things, a very valuable management tool for identifying with staff what they seek to achieve in their work and negotiating with them appropriate objectives and how they will be met. Human beings are generally highly 'goal-seeking', i.e. we identify some things we want (possibly the satisfaction of some needs) and then search for ways to achieve them. The manager can therefore make use of this by exploring the goals with the individual and determining the extent to which work can help to achieve them.

Recognition

Managers quite often take people's work for granted and may fail to acknowledge the everyday contributions that individuals make to the effective running of the organization. If we are busy and running hard to keep up, it is easy to forget the many people who are helping us to make it work. Thus we need to take stock every so often and find genuine ways of acknowledging work well done. The use of staff appraisal or career review, for example, can be a time for a one-to-one exchange about this. It is also a good idea to examine our behaviour in everyday relationships and provide positive feedback where appropriate to individuals.

Team building

Being part of an effective and well-managed team can provide considerable satisfaction for many people, particularly when the team is highly involved in identifying and solving problems and setting their own goals. There has rightly been much emphasis placed on the value of teams and teamwork to achieve results in the public as well as the private sector. Increasingly we need the expertise of a wide range of people to identify and solve the kind of problems that face us in working with patients and clients and for many – particularly those working to an extent autonomously in the community – the team becomes a vital reference point and 'haven' for support.

Equity

In areas such as grades, salary, holiday arrangements, etc., it is important for the manager to be fair and even-handed. Quite often what demotivates a person is not, for example, the salary itself but the salary grade or increase in comparison to that obtained by others who are perceived as doing a similar job. The way in which the organization deals with these issues has to demonstrate a balance between individual needs, about which the manager may know a great deal, with an equitable across-the-board approach which is seen to be fair and not favouring certain individuals. This is a fine balance and needs to be carefully managed.

Appraisal

Appraisal is an increasingly important aspect of any manager's work. A few years ago it was very much limited to the private sector but now it is becoming widespread through the public sector as well and it is important that care is taken in its introduction. Consider the following remarks:

We have to do all these staff appraisals; it'll take ages and ages and I know the staff think it's a waste of their time.

I suppose I'll have to spend the whole of Thursday morning doing staff interviews. Honestly, you'd think the managers would realize we had other more pressing duties. It's just another management chore as far as I'm concerned and the staff feel the same.

Unless care is taken over the way in which an appraisal system is introduced, staff are trained and the system reviewed to ensure that it is working satisfactorily for all parties, then it can easily be seen as 'another chore'. This is a pity, since an effective and respected appraisal system can considerably enhance staff development and contribute to team building and improved morale within the section, ward or department. We aim to provide advice both for those managers who have yet to install a system and for those who have one up and running.

There has always been appraisal in the health service and in social care. It may not have been termed appraisal but most managers have always seen supervision of their staff as part of their responsibilities. This would normally involve keeping an eye open to see how the staff were doing, what progress they were making, where they might be having particular problems and where achieving success.

An effective appraisal system builds on effective supervision. There should be no surprises in an appraisal interview. If the supervision has been good then the issues to be discussed at the appraisal will already be 'on the table' and not sprung on the appraisee who then has to conduct his or her own defence. An appraisal is not a court of law to determine innocence or guilt.

We also need to remember that appraisal does not replace supervision or vice versa; they are complementary processes and the difference between them is that supervision is continuous, whereas appraisal occurs at regular intervals, most often on an annual basis.

Definitions

Appraisal is given different names in different organizations. It can be found under the terms performance review, staff assessment, career review and annual performance interview.

The dictionary definition is: 'An assessment of the worth or quality of a person'. It is a systematic process whereby an individual member of staff has the opportunity to engage in a frank, confidential discussion with his or her manager as to the achievements and shortcoming of the previous 'year'.

There are a number of variants on this theme:

- *Peer appraisal:* This is where a group of colleagues appraise each other.
- *Upward appraisal:* This is where a group of staff appraise their immediate manager.

- *Self appraisal:* This is where the individual is responsible for his or her own appraisal. We will argue that in good systems there is always an element of self appraisal.

The objectives of appraisal

There is little point in setting up an appraisal system or developing one unless the objectives are clear in the minds of all who take part. If these objectives are not clearly indicated to staff then we can get that degree of muddle, grumbling over chores and general disillusionment we saw at the opening of this section. It also represents a considerable waste of staff time and the organization's limited resources.

Appraisal of staff can serve many purposes. In 1977 when appraisal was confined to far fewer organizations and had not been seriously mentioned in the health service or social care, Parkinson (1977) suggested that the objectives of appraisal are:

- to allocate fair and just rewards;
- to identify staff with promotional possibilities;
- to establish a more effective two-way communication system;
- to identify training needs of staff.

Activity

> What do you think should be the objectives of an effective appraisal system with your staff now in the 1990s? Consider this before continuing. Jot down a few ideas, then compare them with ours.

Some of the objectives of effective appraisal today are:

- to provide useful feedback on an individual's performance so as to help current performance;
- to give an opportunity for the appraiser to gain feedback on his/her performance as manager from the appraisee;
- to establish or clarify job descriptions and key results areas;
- to provide a basis for self evaluation;
- to assist in the determination of salaries, financial and other rewards;
- to assist with the clarification of training/staff development needs;
- to discover individual and group needs at work;
- to monitor the effectiveness of procedures and supervision;
- to provide a time for the exchange of ideas, concerns, initiatives; and
- to assist in personnel planning – transfers, promotions, early retirement etc.

The first thing that most people notice on such a list is the mention of 'financial rewards'. We have briefly discussed performance related pay. This is a highly contentious area and, at the time of writing, increasing numbers of

Trusts in the UK are pressing for the right to make local pay awards to staff without being tied to national agreements (Whitley Council and various pay review bodies). There is much pressure against such a move from the various professional associations and unions. We believe that the continued devolution of management responsibilities down to ward and unit level, especially budget responsibility, means that if a member of staff is deemed to be working well above expectations and this becomes apparent from supervision and appraisal, then they should be rewarded differently from another member whose performance is shown to be mediocre.

The question of whether salaries should form part of the appraisal process or not is a difficult one. In the past, especially in the public sector, there was a general view that performance appraisal and pay should not be linked. It was considered that if there was no such direct linkage then staff would be more willing to take part in the appraisal and more likely to speak their minds in an open manner. Increasingly, senior staff in the public sector have had their appraisal and pay linked. This has been partly due to the introduction of short term contracts for senior staff and the negotiation of private sector-type pay agreements linked to performance.

The other contentious issue relating to appraisal is that the system is increasingly being used for 'personnel planning', a term euphemistically used to refer to staff cuts. You could, however, argue that any system of supervision will bring together information which then may be used to inform 'manpower' decisions.

The other items on the list are probably less contentious. Most staff will consider that any kind of appraisal should assist those involved in clarifying their work objectives and any needs for training and development.

You will notice that in this list there is focus on the idea of an *exchange* of ideas. An appraisal should never become an interrogation, with one person doing all the questioning and one doing all the answering. What is needed is a time for open listening.

In Chapter 4 on communications we examined some aspects of Transactional Analysis (TA). It is vital that any appraisal interview should follow the 'adult – adult' tone and not be allowed to slip into the critical parent. If the manager falls into the 'parent' mode, it can easily trigger off a 'crossed transaction' so that the interview ends up as a disagreeable squabble.

Appraisals can easily be seen as unfair, as a system imposed by authorities on individuals. It is crucial to establish the right attitude to the process.

Establishing the right atmosphere

All staff should ideally be involved in the development, maintenance and evaluation of the appraisal system. It should not be a top-down, imposed system.

- All staff must be appraised. It is very important that no senior staff are seen to 'escape' the process.

- Appraisees must really understand what is being asked of them when they are appraised.
- Appraisers must also know fully what is being asked of them when they are asked to carry out appraisal interviews.
- The criteria on which staff are to be appraised should be open and must be related to actual work carried out. There should be no reference to personal traits, likes and dislikes.
- The appraisee should be in a position to question or challenge comments made in the appraisal.
- All those involved in appraisals should have access to training.
- There should be opportunities for follow-up training and staff development.
- The appraisal system should be subject to review.

Different forms of appraisal.

We mentioned earlier that although manager-subordinate appraisal was by far the most common, there are other forms. There are a number of instances reported in the *Health Services Journal* of hospitals where staff are starting to *upward appraise* their managers. This practice has been in place in some service sector organizations for the last decade. At first such a practice can be threatening to managers (Hart, 1994).

At one hospital where it has proved successful an outsider was brought in to chair the appraisal and act as 'referee'; this helped to reduce any possible friction and unease. Questionnaires were issued to all staff and completed anonymously. The results were summarized and fed back to the managers.

As with many such innovations the important thing is to learn from experience and seek to build a system which all staff find helpful. The first time this system was tried, the 'referee' talked with all the staff and then fed the results back to the manager. After this meeting there was a whole staff gathering to air the results. This was considered by the author of the article to have been the most useful aspect of the whole process.

Some organizations are running group appraisals. For example, in the voluntary sector teams are sometimes encouraged to assess their experience when a particular project has been completed rather than simply at the end of each year. These assessments are put together as a team effort. The results are summarized and sent to the team manager who then in an informal meeting discusses the outcomes with the group and together they agree on future key areas for development, training, etc.

The questions members of the group might ask themselves could include:

- In what areas could we improve our practice?
- Looking at the skills/experience mix of the present team, what training/ staff development, secondment, etc. would be helpful to the way the group could operate in the future?

As team work and the importance of team building is emphasized, such peer group appraisal would appear to be of increasing importance in the health service and social care.

Conducting the appraisal interview

We examined various aspects of interviewing in Chapter 4; we again emphasize that it is very important that the interview is planned carefully and carried out with the greatest care and respect for both parties.

The process can be divided into three parts: *before, during* and *afterwards*. Let us state each in turn.

Before

Plenty of warning must be given to those involved in the appraisal. The interview should be based on the concept of negotiation, that is both 'sides' should come equally prepared and ready for a 'win/win' process (*see* Chapter 7). If one party to the interview is unprepared, caught off-guard by the questions, made to feel like a child by an inquisition, then this balance cannot be maintained and one side will have the advantage. Part of any such warning will be the way in which the appraisal forms are distributed. Staff must have sufficient time to gather their thoughts, talk with colleagues including those in a supervisory capacity, and complete the form so as to give plenty of time for the appraiser to read it.

During

It is very important that any interview has some kind of structure, none more so than the appraisal. We would suggest the following pattern:

- Make certain that the purpose of the interview is well understood. This is particularly important if staff are new and experiencing their first appraisal.
- Explain the procedures. Outline briefly how the interview will proceed. Clarify agendas. Ask what topics the appraisee wants to cover, then go over any you feel should be included.
- Review previous appraisal, the actions agreed, commitments made together with existing job description, in particular any key results areas targeted from the previous appraisal.
- Review any comments on performance made by supervisors.
- Review the way the appraiser has been managed over the past year. This is to provide feedback for the manager.
- Discuss topics raised by both appraisee and appraiser from the agenda agreed on earlier. Focus on any training/staff development needs.

- Agree on actions to be taken by whom and by when to achieve agreed objectives/key results areas.
- Deal with any other business – matters not dealt with, ideas for progress.
- Summarize; check back for mutual understanding.

Activity

Let us see what can actually happen . Read the following dialogue and then jot down what advice you would give to the manager conducting this appraisal interview.

The scene is the manager's office in a residential nursing home. Mary, an auxiliary nurse, is due to enter for her annual appraisal.

Manager: Hullo Mary, do come in. Sit down. Fine. Now we're both very busy and I don't want to keep you longer than is necessary. I see from my notes that it's almost eighteen months since we last had an appraisal. Never mind. I'm sure we'll be able to catch up. How've you been doing? Could I start by asking you if your job has changed much since we had this last appraisal?

Mary: No not much, pretty well the same. Just getting busier.

Manager: Well, can we look at what your supervisor has said about your work.

Mary: She's never said anything to me against my work.

Manager: No well in general she's very happy with your work. She says your time keeping has been excellent.

Mary: Oh I'm never late and I've only been off with the flu.

Manager: Yes that's very good; however she also says that at times you have been rather grumpy with patients and that she has had to remind you about this on several occasions. What do you say to that?

Mary: I don't think that's fair. I just happen to have had a couple of difficult patients.

Manager: Well she says something more than that. She says that it is your attitude which at times lets you down.

Mary: Well I don't agree. I like my job.

Manager: I don't think that's the issue at stake, it's a question of attitudes. The way in which you relate to patients.

Mary: Well this comes as a bit of a shock. I thought everyone was happy with my work.

Manager: Now don't get me wrong Mary. I'm not saying that there's anything wrong with your work...

Mary :   But you've just said I'm grumpy to patients.

Manager: Could you let me finish. Your supervisor says that your work is fine. That you come in on time and put in a full day. You keep your area very clean and tidy and all the beds are properly made. Generally you appear to get on well with the patients.

Mary: But I'm grumpy.

Manager. No not to all, just on occasions to a few. It's this point Mary that we have to address. Do you accept that fact that you have been grumpy.

Mary: Well we all have our bad days. (*This discussion continues for some time*)

Manager: Could we now move on. Is there anything you would like to raise with me?

Mary: No.

Manager: Do you have any training needs?

Mary: What sort of training?

Manager: Well I'm just going through this list. Training?

Mary: Can't think of anything.

Manager: Is there anything else you'd like to raise at this interview?

Mary: Well I haven't really thought. You see I only got warning of this interview yesterday. I can't think of anything just now.

Manager: Right. Well to summarize. You agree that your attitude with some patients has not been 100 per cent and that you're going to try harder in this direction. You're going to try to be a little more cheerful with some of the patients, particularly the ones in the annexe. You could see no training needs at present. Well thank you very much for coming. I've enjoyed talking to you. If there's anything you remember that you wanted to bring up do let me know.

There are a number of issues here. This is not a very *productive* interview. It is what too many appraisals can become, that is a charade. The appraiser has all the cards and the appraisee tries to see what lies beneath them.

There has been a *lack of real preparation*. Mary had not thought of the issues. She had not been helped to consider her agenda. Many staff need such coaching from their supervisors and team. There is little point in asking if someone needs any training unless he or she has had time and possibly assistance to think through the issue; to reflect on performance; to be made familiar with what training actually means, how accessible it might be and whether it is pitched at an appropriate level.

There is very little *structure* to this interview. The opening is rushed: 'both very busy', could be read by the appraisee as 'can only give you a few minutes'. It is important at the start to signify that there is time available and that there will be no interruptions. This is 'quality' time whereby the appraisee can have their manager's committed attention. The start of the interview is also the time to fully clarify the agenda. You notice how the word 'training' jumped out at Mary. She is immediately defensive, suspecting probably that there is a hidden agenda here. The supervisor's report similarly springs out as a threat.

The *conclusion is similarly rushed*. It is very important to gain both under-standing and mutual commitment to a programme of action or key results areas.

The whole *tone* of this interview is, in TA terms, very 'parent–child'. It is an exercise in discipline and control rather than in negotiation and arriving at an understanding.

Afterwards

It is all to easy to lose sight of the fact that appraisal interviews need to be followed up. Staff rightly get upset and disappointed when various short and long term promises and commitments are entered into at the interview ('I'll see your supervisor this week', or 'I shall insist you attend that course at the end of the month' etc.) and then nothing happens. There must be follow-up and it must be communicated to the appraisee.

This then takes us back to where we started: that appraisal is but part of a general programme of supervision. It is there to allow the growth and development of all staff in the organization. For that reason it deserves to be taken seriously; that means resources and time need to be devoted to it. In answer to those grumbles we quoted at the start, a whole morning given up to listening to staff during perhaps two or three appraisals should be a very good investment.

Training your staff

Your appraisal system should assist you as manager in identifying training needs amongst your staff – that is one very good reason for having such a system. However evidence should also be available from other sources, such as:

- a training needs analysis (TNA), i.e. a systematic audit of training needs, sometimes carried out by external facilitators using a variety of methodologies: observation, work analysis, including comparisons of job descriptions with actual duties, questionnaires, interviews, focused groups, etc. (Like the communication audit mentioned on page 106 it seeks to establish a baseline on which decisions about training can be made.);
- general supervision;
- information from patient feedback/surveys/complaints and suggestions;
- evidence from audits – external and internal;
- general observation, impressions from other managers, supervisors;
- self assessment – individuals' own views as to their training needs;
- peer group assessments: the team itself suggesting the most effective training for its members;
- comparisions made from 'benchmarking' your organization with others;
- comments assessments from courses staff have been on, etc.

Having got the evidence from any or all of these sources, decisions then have to be made in the light of the available budget for training as to how the money should be spent. We have already identified both mentoring and coaching as extremely important complements to a training plan. The question is what should you put alongside them. We suggest you should consider these questions when selecting from various training plans:

- Does the training seek to explore the individuals' attitudes and expectations in relation to the programme? (If it operates on the surface and never seeks to engage people then there will be little if any 'buying in' to what the trainers say. This will result in 'surface' learning; engagement only at a superficial level with little or no change in behaviours.)
- Do those who carry out the training make use of examples, case studies directly related to the trainees' work experience?
- Does the training offered fit into some kind of plan – both from the individual's point of view and for his or her unit/team?
- Does the training hook into what the trainee already knows and seek to build on this knowledge? The danger if it does not is that it can de-skill and demotivate the individual.
- Does the training offer feedback on performance of the trainee as he or she passes through the various stages? Is this feedback easily understood?
- Are there opportunities in the training for there to be some consolidation of skill and knowledge?
- Does the training offer a variety of learning strategies (remember Honey and Mumford in our introduction)? There is considerable evidence that we have different learning styles and a programme that does not cater for this variety will not be successful with many who attend.

We would add, again with reference back to our introduction, that the manager must try to create and sustain a 'learning climate' within the organization. One very important factor in this is the attention that is given to people who receive training. All too often people return to work after a course and their experience is given hardly a mention, in fact there is often expressed resentment at their having been away 'having an easy time'. It must be said that there are many staff and not a few managers who think of training very much as rewards and therefore those who do not get picked to go are deemed not be worthy in some way. Hence it is not surprising that these attitudes should prevail.

Encourage staff who have been on courses to report back; to circulate their ideas and handouts; encourage them to present or write and so circulate projects carried out from their studies. As a manager make sure that you see them, talk to them and see what lessons can be learned.

Conclusion

Your *direct* interest in staff development as expressed through a good selection and recruitment policy, an approach to induction which welcomes new staff to their posts, the setting up of coaching and mentoring schemes that support staff, and the development of a non-threatening and productive appraisal system will pay very real dividends in *making the best of your staff.*

References

Hart J (1994) The only way is up. *Health Services Journal,* 14 March.
Maslow A H (1954) *Motivation and Personality.* Harper & Row, New York.
Parkinson R (1977) *Personnel Management* 9 (11), 31–8.

Further reading

Ellis R J and McClintock A (1994) *If You Take My Meaning.* Edward Arnold, London.
Goodworth C T (1985) *Effective Interviewing.* Business Books, London.
Graham H T (1991) *Human Resource Management.* Pitman, London.
Statt D (1994) *Psychology at Work.* Macmillan, London.

15

Conclusion

The subtitle of this book is 'A Guide to Self-development', and we hope that as you have read it through and considered the case studies and checklists that you have felt just a little more 'developed' as a manager than when you started out. In mentioning case studies we emphasized in our introduction the importance of reflection on experience, and the integration of theory to practice. Now having read the book, we urge you to go on reflecting and making these links between your work as a manager and the various theories and approaches we have outlined.

Perhaps, with some justification, you feel a little overwhelmed at all the things that managers have to understand and be competent in; perhaps you feel that it is not a piece of PIE after all. But do not feel that you should implement the various lessons here all in one go. First consider how you manage yourself – your time, energy, learning, staff colleagues and bosses. One practical result that we hope comes from reading this book is that you will be able to clarify your role with your own line manager and then do the same with colleagues and staff. So many of the problems we identified in our case studies came about because of a lack of role definition. Just think how much better life would have been for Lottie if she had these issues resolved. Secondly, see which of these areas is a priority for you and your staff. Try to plan out a strategy of review and then implementation. Link your reading with such a review.

You will find that some of the chapters in the book seem to contain more concrete details of 'how to do' things. You may have noticed that this is because some of the issues that we have introduced and discussed are more conceptually based than others. The way you choose to communicate or lead or team build are very dependent on your own preferred style. There are key issues to consider and some good principles to follow, but as with learning style, ways of communicating or leading are personal and reflect much of our characteristics as individuals. Contrast this with setting standards, time management or costing. These are quite tangible and pragmatic skills. There are some right and wrong ways of going about them. You will find therefore that these chapters contain 'easier' or more concrete information with less choices to be made but more work to be done.

Some of these key links we feel we should emphasize are as follows:

- Change within the health and social care service will go as rapidly as now. Managers have to 'keep fit' for these changes. Continual self development will be one of the keys to such a keep fit programme. This book and the follow-up reading is but a part of such a programme. Negotiate and advocate a keep fit programme for yourself and others you are working with. Examine your own training and staff development record. Consider those areas where you feel you need further help and advice. Remember that attendance on a course is only one way of reaching your goal. See who can do some coaching for you, find out where 'they do it better' – benchmarking – and go and learn. Be open to learning new ways when you are not within your normal work situation: keep your eyes open for good practice in any area of retail, service, recreation and leisure industries. It is amazing how many good ways there are of doing what you do – serving the customer.

- Change has to be managed; it just cannot be left to chance and whim. Staff being the most precious resource of any health or social care service, the way in which they are managed during times of turbulence is critical for morale, for the service they offer and thus ultimately to patient and client welfare. We have pointed up some methods for managing change. Communication and information are often the keys: listening to others and their fears, doubts and ideas, communicating openly about the need for change, providing a reasoned case and reviewing the change. Everyone who goes along with change should be promised some kind of review of its progress.

- Devolved power in some form or other is another powerful form of change and is here to stay. Increasingly, managers will have to cope with delegation of their authority to staff. This will not be easy. Some staff will accuse you of dumping, some will relish the challenge. The manager will increasing have to be prepared to coach his or her staff into their new roles. Delegation is one skill that we can guarantee will be more and more important for all managers in health and social care. If you have not done much, start practising. Remember the advice: 'keep your eyes wide open but your hands off.' Do not cut adrift with no lifeboat. Stay in touch but do not smother, and remember what is plain sense to you may seem very puzzling to the person asked to do the job. So brief clearly and if necessary re-brief.

- Leadership will increasingly mean working with teams and all the necessary skills in building up and maintaining the team. It looks as though teams will need to become more flexible; that means considerations of skills mix and with it more serious consideration of training and staff development for the team not just the individuals within it. Think about the message from Belbin and how people play two roles: their technical and their team role. Try out a little Belbin type analysis of the various team types you have. Perhaps you will need to import a 'plant'.

- Increasingly, managers in health and social care will have to think of standards and contracts and these contracts will have standards on which they are based. This implies a knowledge of how standards are reached, an ability to negotiate and communicate these standards with staff and colleagues. The development of tables of performance will probably continue and make managers' work more available to scrutiny. If managers do not push for qualitative standards and examine ways within their areas of responsibility that quality can be measured then they will often be stuck with the rather crude quantitative measures that their managers impose on them. Start collecting the data. Encourage all your staff to do the same. Keep records of improvements. Work your data up for presentation. If you do not someone else will collect it and present it for you and that may be hard to swallow.

- Accountability in terms of resources will also be an ever increasing feature of life for managers. It will no longer be enough to consider finance and budgeting as something that others do, for you and to you. It is a process, no matter how junior a manager you feel yourself to be, that you will have to be able to take informed decisions on and ask informed questions of those who are the 'experts'. Take out your phrase book and learn the vocabulary of costs, budgets and financial measurement; know something about fixed and variable cost, apportionment and zero budgeting. If you do it will mean that you will be in a better position to negotiate.

- Negotiation is a key word for managers, a word that has occurred very often in this text. Remember, if you 'don't ask, you won't get'. You will need to negotiate for more time, more resources, more equipment, more staff and that will only come about with negotiation. And negotiation means having a case prepared. This is why an appreciation of costing is so import. Prepare a good case, communicate it clearly and be prepared to listen to the other side's worries and doubts, so that you can move towards a win/win situation.

- Time is one of the most important resources – particularly your time. If you have not already done so, take a very hard look at the present way you spend your time and think how, as a precious resource, it could be better spent. Think how your staff spend their time. Bring them into time management. Coach them in more effective ways of using time. Coach them in the difference between 'efficient' and 'effective' and between 'urgent' and 'important'.

- Poor communications are at the heart of many problems within health and social care. Carry out a communications audit of your section, ward, unit or department. Try to track exactly where the communication goes to and who receives it – or fails to. An audit can discover some of these problems, but remember that often it is not just about channels and systems but about attitudes and expectations of those communicating one to another. Tease out the expectations and the attitudes. Clarify individual roles as sender and receiver. Remember to avoid the 'dwindle' factor – if you start a staff news-sheet do not drop it after two editions.

- Communication will increasingly mean making use of technology and the various electronic means that we can use to communicate with one another. Despite all the advances that faxing, internets and video conferencing offer, the need, however, will often be for better and more regular face-to-face communication with staff and colleagues and with your line managers, to say nothing of patients.

- The need to change attitudes and culture at work will always be a challenge to managers and will often entail conflict. Remember that some conflict is healthy; the crucial skill is to be able to move from conflict to consensus. Here the individual manager's own interpersonal skills and style of managing are crucial. How is your bicycle: the one with three gears or the one with twenty three? Reflect on the way you currently ride. Are you using the most modern? Do you have enough range? Appropriate is a word that has echoed throughout this text. We have referred to it in talking about management and leadership style – the direct through to the collaborative. Be conscious of your own style. Appropriate means an ability to judge from the situation and the characters involved what is the best course of action – or inaction.

Before we finish our thoughts on self development for managers, go back to the learning styles that were mentioned in the first chapter – the introduction. Think of the things that you have tried to work on during the course of using this book and work out whether you have been a pragmatist, activist, theorist or reflector. Have you been a pragmatist on costing and a theorist on communications? Whichever way you have tried to assimilate this information, remember that others have varying styles of comprehension and you should try to encourage people in accordance with their preferred mode of learning. We are all different and perhaps the key to a really good manager is the ability to recognize this and work with it to make a cohesive and effective team offering the best level of service possible.

We hope this book has assisted you and will go on assisting you in the search for that correct judgement.

Index